HIV/AIDS PREVENTION EDUCATION FOR EDUCATIONAL INSTITUTIONS

INTERNATIONAL ENCYCLOPAEDIA OF AIDS - 9

HIV/AIDS
PREVENTION EDUCATION FOR EDUCATIONAL INSTITUTIONS

Editor

Dr. Digumarti Bhaskara Rao

M.Sc., M.A., M.A., M.Ed., Ph.D.

Dean, Faculty of Education

Member, Academic Senate

Ex-Chairman, Board of Studies in Education

Member, Research Advisory Committee

Acharya Nagarjuna University

D-43, S.V.N. Colony

Guntur - 522 006 (India)

DPH

DISCOVERY PUBLISHING HOUSE PVT. LTD.

NEW DELHI-110 002

First Published - 2000

Reprinted - 2015

ISBN: 978-81-7141-465-9 (Set)

ISBN: 978-81-7141-531-1

HIV/AIDS Prevention Education for Educational Institutions

Published by:

DISCOVERY PUBLISHING HOUSE PVT. LTD.
4383/4B, Ansari Road, Darya Ganj
New Delhi-110 002 (India)
Phone: +91-11-23279245, 43596064-65
Fax: +91-11-23253475
E-mail: discoverypublishinghouse@gmail.com
sales@discoverypublishinggroup.com
web: www.discoverypublishinggroup.com

Printed at:
Infinity Imaging Systems
Delhi

PREFACE

The HIV/AIDS is a new phenomenon in the human society. HIV destroys the immune system of human individuals, producing a defenselessness fatal state known as AIDS. The World Health Organisation has estimated that already one in every two hundred and fifty adults in the world is infected with Human Immunodeficiency Virus and according to WHO's projections a total of forty million men women and children worldwide will have been infected with HIV by the turn of this twentieth century. Visualising the devastating effects of the HIV/AIDS epidemic within our life times and beyond is difficult. Probably, no other disease in recent times has had the impact on human society generated by HIV/AIDS.

The HIV/AIDS epidemic has brought into focus many health related ethical, legal and human rights issues. This epidemic requires immediate and effective responses in new programming areas: attitudinal and behavioural changes, community-based care and support initiatives, and the maintenance of human development in the face of increasing rates of illness and deaths. At this point, education enters the scene as it can alter the HIV/AIDS situation since it brings change in the behaviour of the people.

This *International Encyclopaedia of AIDS* presents the worldwide information about HIV/AIDS, issues and challenges, reports and reviews, ethics laws and human rights, and educational activities and programmes to keep the policy makers, planners, professionals, activists, researchers, educationists, teachers and students well informed of the epidemic.

Dr. Digumarti Bhaskara Rao
26 January 1999
The Republic Day of India

ACKNOWLEDGEMENT

I am thankful to the World Health Organisation and its associated offices for using their material namely School Health Education to prevent AIDS and STD: A Resource Package for Curriculum Planners-Handbook for Curriculum Planners. Student's Activities, Teachers' Guide, Global Programme on AIDS-HIV Prevention and Care: Teaching Modules for Nurses and Midwives, Global Programme on AIDS. Community HIV Prevention Handbook; STD care Management-workbooks 1-7, Facing the Challenge of HIV/ AIDS STDs: A Gender-based Response; HIV/AIDS and STD surveillance Data Management and Use-Report, Bangkok, 1995; Carrying out HIV Sentinal Surveillance-A Guide for Programme Managers, AIDS Prevention and Care in the workplace: Enhancing the Role of Private Sector; HIV Testing Policies and Guidelines; Carrying out HIV Sentinel surveillance; AIDS Prevention; Understanding and Living with AIDS; AIDS: A Modern Epidemic; HIV/AIDS in South-East Asia: IXth meeting of the National Programme Managers, New Delhi, 1993; Information, Education and Communication: A Guide for AIDS Programme Managers, Handbook on AIDS Home Care; HIV/AIDS in South-East Asia: A Pictorial summary; etc.

I am thankful to the United Nations Development Programme, UNDP's HIV and Development Programme, and UNDP's Regional Projects on HIV and Development for using their material namely Economic Implications of AIDS in Asia; Socio Economic Implications of the Epidemic; NGOs Working with Sex workers; NGO Responses to HIV/AIDS in Asia-Case Studies; HIV in the Workplace: Dealing with the Issues-Role Plays, Development and the HIV Epidemic, Law Ethics and HIV; HIV Law and Law Reform; Issue Papers; Study Papers; Working Papers; etc.

I am thankful to the Health and Nutrition Centre, Republic of Philippines for using its material namely sourcebook on HIV/AIDS Prevention Education for Tertiary Educational Institutions.

I am thankful to the Curriculum Development Programme, Ministry of Education, Government of Thailand for using its material namely Institutional Modules for AIDS Education.

I am thankful to US Department of Health and Human Services: Whitman-Walker Clinic, Inc., USA; East-West Centre, USA; National AIDS Control Organisation, Government of India; Academy of Culture Communication Education Science and Service, Guntur, United Nations and its agencies for using their material.

I am grateful to Bhaskar Bhattacharji; V. Alexeev, Geeta Sethi, Elizabeth Reid, Mina Mauerstein-Bail, A. A. Trinidad, Palomi Cuchi, D. Pushpa Latha for their kind co-operation.

Dr. Digumarti Bhaskara Rao,
Secretary
ACCESS
D-43, S.V. N. Colony,
Guntur-522 006

CONTENTS

1

PROGRAMMED INSTRUCTION

BACKGROUND INFORMATION ABOUT AIDS

Note To The Teacher

The historical background as well as statistical data (e.g, pie and bar graphs) on the incidence and spread of HIV/AIDS will be presented to introduce this lesson. These statistical data will serve as evidence of the seriousness of this disease as well as highlight the current and future risks of contracting HIV infection

Early Beginnings of AIDS

AIDS was first discovered in 1981 in the United States. Studies show that the disease was uncommon until the late 1970's and early 1980's when more cases began to be seen in both Central Africa and the United States. The disease has now spread and is continuing to spread to most countries of the world.

In Africa, about the same number of men and women have AIDS. In the United States and Europe, the disease was first seen among men who had sex with other men. Now, in Europe and the United States, AIDS has also spread among men and women of heterosexual relations. In the East, AIDS cases have also been found among people who share hypodermic needles to inject drugs.

In Asian countries like the Philippines, some cases of AIDS were due to the transfusion of blood infected with HIV, mother to child during pregnancy, at birth, or shortly after birth (pre-natal, natal and perinatal) Figure 1 shows the cause of HIV infections by mode of transmission from 1984 to April 1994.

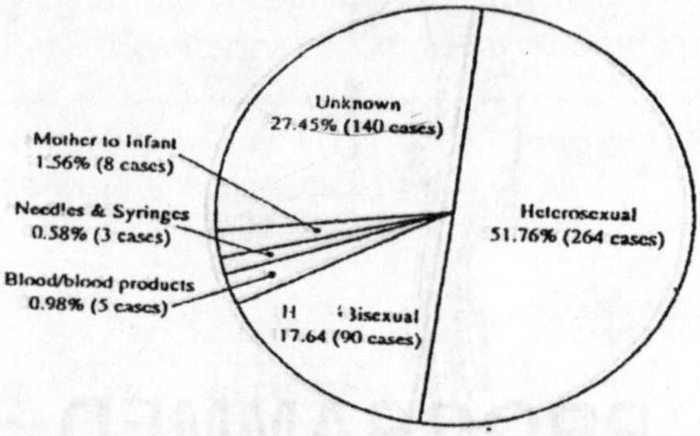

Figure 1. Cause of HIV Infection by Mode of Transmission

The percentage of HIV infection by mode of transmission from 1984 to present is presented in Figure 2.

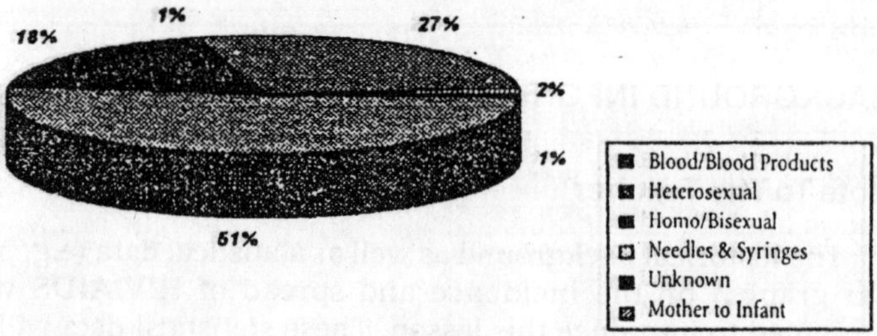

Figure 2. Percentage of HIV Infection by Mode of Transmission, 1984-1994.

Figure 2 shows the cumulative HIV/AIDS cases as of April 1994 reflecting the continuous increase in the number of cases.

Cause of AIDS

AIDS is caused by a virus that is too tiny to be seen by the naked eye called Human-Immuno-deficiency Virus (HIV).

Once HIV enters the body, it lives and grows in the blood cells and body fluids of the infected person.

This virus is a retrovirus which infects the white blood cells, specifically the T4 helper cell which usually fights off infection of the human body.

Human blood contains different groups of cells that play a major role in the defense against disease. One group of these cells called lymphocytes includes B cells and several types of T cells. The B cells produce important infection fighting chemical compounds called antibodies. Helper "T" cells assist B cells to produce antibodies that fight invading disease causing germs such as viruses.

In a person with HIV infection/AIDS, the HIV infects and kills helper cells. This phenomenon makes the immune system weak and is eventually destroyed. This deterioration or destruction of the immune system renders the body increasingly vulnerable to attack by other viruses, fungi, protozoa and bacteria, which ultimately results in death.

Clinical Manifestation of HIV Infection/AIDS

Infection with HIV may cause various kinds of sickness. The infection first shows itself through mild signs of illness. This stage may be followed by more serious ailments. Finally, the infected person may become very weak and suffer from dangerous, often unusual forms of sickness. AIDS develops in this last stage of infection with the virus.

The spectrum of HIV infection: .

1. *HIV Asymptomatic.* This applies to those people who show evidence of HIV infection only through laboratory testing. Examples of these are those people whose blood tests are "positive" for antibodies of HIV and look healthy and well.

A positive HIV antibody blood test means one has been exposed to the HIV virus and can infect other people.

But a positive result does not tell you whether one has AIDS. At present, it is thought that only some of those exposed to the virus will develop AIDS.

2. *HIV symptomatic.* This refers to those people who have developed a mild form of the disease with symptoms such as unexplained weight loss, enlarged glands, night sweats which persist for three (3) months or more and neurologic symptoms which are manifested as memory loss and other impairments.

3. *AIDS.* This refers to the people whose HIV infection has developed into AIDS. The immune system is impaired and the person has one or more opportunistic infections/malignancies.

Among the common illnesses seen are: a) Kaposi's sarcoma (KS); b) Pneumocystis carinii pneumonia (PCP).

Pneumocystis carnii pneumonia is a lung infection caused by a protozoa Pneumocystis carnii. Severe immune deficiency or malnutrition allows the organism to multiply in the lungs gradually filling them with pneumocysts.

Kaposi's sarcoma is a form of cancer or tumor of the blood vessel walls.

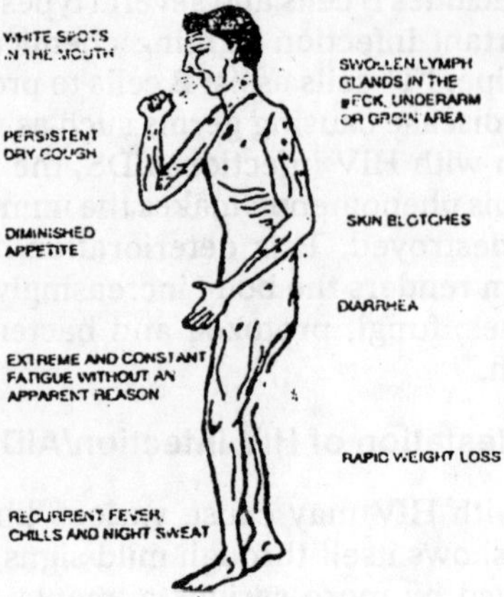

Figure 3 shows the picture of a man manifesting the various symptoms of AIDS.

- Constitutional symptoms, particularly over a period exceeding a few days, may be due to HIV disease These include unexplained fatigue or tiredness, malaise, anorexia, weight loss and fever and sweats.
- Skin complaints are common including skin blotches, seborrhoeic dermatitis, eczema, folliculitis, herpes complex and fungal infections including those affecting the nails
- Gastrointestinal symptoms are common in HIV infection/AIDS disease, but are often non-specific with occasional mild diarrhea, over a period of several months.
- Respiratory symptoms such as persistent dry cough, increasing shortness of breath for several weeks Examination may reveal weight loss or other signs of HIV disease (oral hairy leukoplakia, oral thrush)
- Central nervous system symptoms include headache, visual disturbance (scotoma, blurred vision), paraesthesiae, vomiting and fits.

Mode of Transmission of AIDS Virus

Everyone who has been infected with HIV can pass the virus to someone else. HIV has been shown to be transmitted through three modes. (Refer to Figure 1.)

1. Sexual contact

HIV is passed from one person to another through sexual contact where there is exchange of semen or vaginal and other body (blood) fluids. Unconventional sexual activity such as anal oral contact can spread the HIV virus and is therefore dangerous.

So far, the greatest number of cases of HIV infection/ AIDS occurs as a result of sexual transmission. The infection can be passed from a man to a woman, from a woman to a man (Heterosexuals) and between members of the same sex (Homosexuals).

If you choose to have sex with several partners (multiple partners), you increase the risk of becoming infected by each partner you have. However, it is not just a question of how many partners you have. Any one act of unprotected sex with a person who is infected with HIV could result in you becoming infected.

2. Exposure to infected blood and blood products

a. Sharing Needles

HIV can be passed by sharing needles which contain infected blood. Considering that by injecting into the vein, drug users draw blood up into the needle and syringe, sharing needles becomes a very risky activity which has caused many cases of HIV infection.

Any used needle that has not been properly sterilized can carry the virus from an infected person to the next user of the needle. It does not matter what the syringe contains. The risk is from the infected blood contaminating the needle and syringe.

Needles and knives used for tattoos, for scarring the face and body and for traditional medicine can also pass on HIV if they are not properly sterilized before use on each person. It is always wise to remember that HIV can be passed from one person to another through infected blood left on instruments used in activities mentioned above. Tools used for any procedure that cuts the skin should be sterilized before each use.

b. Transfusion with unscreened/infected blood

Another way HIV can be transmitted other than sex is through infected blood. For example, blood used for transfusions, when obtained from a person carrying HIV, can pass the infection to the person receiving that blood. Receiving blood transfusion of blood not screened for HIV poses a potential risk for contracting the virus. However, one cannot get HIV infection from giving blood if the blood taking equipment is sterilized.

At the start of the HIV infection, the danger of infected blood was not known. Now that it is proven that blood used for medical purposes may have been infected with HIV, many countries have initiated programs to test these blood supplies and dispose of all infected blood. Increasingly, blood is being tested for HIV worldwide. If you are not sure whether the blood is tested in your area, inquire from the proper authority such as the Philippine National Red Cross, the Department of Health and other accredited blood centers.

3. An HIV positive pregnant woman

If a woman is infected with HIV, she can infect her child during pregnancy, childbirth or after birth. Researches revealed that 30 to 40% of babies born to women infected with HIV will be born infected. These children usually do not live long. An HIV positive woman who is considering pregnancy needs to consult or seek advise from doctor or trained health personnel who are authorities on the risks of the disease .

PREVENTIVE MEASURES

HIV infection/AIDS can be prevented through the following:

1. Responsible sexual behaviour

Some behaviour is likely to put a person at greater risk of HIV infection Hence, people should avoid:'

a. having sex with multiple sexual partners or
b. having sex with persons who have sex with multiple partners
c. alcoholism and drug abuse which can lead to irresponsible sexual behaviour

2. Screening of blood for transfusion

We have learned earlier that transfusion of unscreened blood can transn HIV. So blood must be screened for HIV before transfusion.

3. Avoiding sharing of needles

Needles should never be shared and need to be sterilized. However, since sterilization would require continuous boiling of 30 to 45 minutes and proper storage, use of new and disposable needles and syringes for every injection is recommended. Shared needles should be immediately dropped into canisters which can be sealed. Sterilizing needles by boiling for 20 minutes is good and safe practice. Disposable needles can also be used if one can afford to do so.

4. Preventing pregnancy if the mother is HIV positive

An HIV positive woman should seek professional help or counsel prior to getting pregnant.

5. Maintaining good health and healthy habits

An HIV infected individual who continues to practice good health and healthy habits will have more chances of delaying the onset of AIDS.

6. Disseminating information about AIDS

At present, AIDS has no known cure. Education is considered to be the most effective strategy to prevent this pandemic disease. Hopefully through the educative process, scientific knowledge, desirable attitudes and healthy practices related to HIV prevention must be developed and internalized by the population, particularly the students and other vulnerable groups.

TEACHERS GUIDE ON AIDS PREVENTION EDUCATION FOR EDUCATIONAL INSTITUTION

Objectives	Concepts	Suggested Activities	Evaluation	Reference
Upon completion of the lesson, the student is able to:				
1. Identify the causative agent AIDS	1. Everybody should know about AIDS 1.2 AIDS is caused by a virus called Human Immuno-Deficiency Virus (HIV) 1.2.1 The virus infects the white blood cells which normally fights infection. 1.3 AIDS is a fatal disease that has no known cure yet.	Lecture/discussion with visuals on the virus causing AIDS Programmed Instruction Learning Module 1 Cause and Effects of AIDS	Paper-and-pencil test	UNESCO Proap, Adolescent Education: Sexually Transmitted Disease, Module 1 (Bangkok: UNESCO PROAP, 1991)p.9 of AIDS
2. Describe the clinical manifestations of AIDS	2. AIDS is acquire, it is not hereditary. 2.1 The spectrum of HIV Infection includes:HIV asymptomatic-Those who show evidence of HIV infection only through laboratory testing, i.e., those people whose blood tests "positive" for antibodies of HIV and are well. HIV symptomatic-Those who are HIV and antibody positive and who have developed a mild form of the disease with symptoms such as unexplained weight loss, enlarged glands, night sweats which persist	—do—		WHO/UNESCO, Education to Prevent AIDS/STD in the Pasific (Paris: WHO/UNESCO, 1991), pp. 10-11.

	for 3 months or more, and neurologic symptoms which are manifested as memory loss and other impairments. AIDS diagnosed-Those peoople suffering from fully developed AIDS symptoms. The immune system is impaired and the person has one or more opportunistic infections.			
3. Explain the psychosocial/	3. AIDS affects the individual, the family, community and the nation as a whole. Emotional impact of AIDS on the individual; 1. Fear 2. Anxiety 3. Anger 4. Hopelessness 5. Loss of Self-esteem *Social Impact* 1. Isolation/discrimination 2. Stigma 3. Disruption of family solidarity *Economical* 1. Economic dislocation due to disruption of employment opportunity 2. Expenses due to prolonged hospitalization The HIV carrier should be responsible enough to seek counselling and treatment from any available heatlh personal in the community.	Panel Discussion on issues re: Impact of AIDS on the individual, family and community Film showing if school has available facilities	A critique on the Panel Discussion on film showing Graded observation, by using rating scale Submission of report on the socio-moral and economical effects of AIDS on the individual the national and international impact of AIDS to economic development	Adrian Mcss, ed., HIV and AIDS Management (Oxford: Oxford University Press, 1992), pp. 63-74. Submission of eassay on
4. Demonstrate beginning skills in counselling persons with AIDS	4. Persons with AIDS should be accorded humane and compasionate treatment by the community. The	Socio Drama "Counselling a person with HIV/AIDS"	Graded observation based on criteria set by the teacher	Basic books on counseling teachnique being in

Objectives	Concepts	Suggested Activities	Evaluation	Reference
	should be helped, trained and supported towards a decent livelihood, recreation and formation of self-help groups.		(Observation Checklist	the course
5. List down government and non-government health agencies in the community where persons infected with HIV/AIDS may be helped	5. There are government and non-government organization which have special services for people with HIV/AIDS.	Preparation of survey instrument and conduct survey using the prepared instrument.	Grade according to criteria in the submitted accomplished survey form	Good and Seates, criteria Method of Research (New York: McGraw Hill Books Co. 1989) pp.
6. Discuss preventive measures to incidence of AIDS	6. Practices to prevent AIDS. 1. screening of blood for transfusion 2. avoiding sharing of infected 3. Information/Education and values education	Programmed Instruction Learning Module III AIDS & Its Prevention	Attitude Scale Simulation of selected selected cases application to target clientele	University of the Phlippines, College of Education, RD Committee, Mannual of Education Research (Quezon City: RD Committee, 19—/, pp. 14-15, 22-23.
	Behaviour that help prevent AIDS 1. The formation fo good habits, Correct attitudes, values and behaviour towards sex and sexuality will help prevent HIV/AIDS infection. These can eventually lead to a more productive and satisfying life.	Case study-factual or hypothetial Mini-survey on Sexual Behaviour Risks/Practices of college students using Focused Group Discussion	Graded-analysis of cases presented	UNESCO PROAP, Adolescent Education: Sexually Transmitted Diseases, Module IV (Bangkok: UNESCO, PPOAP, 1991), P-26. WHO/UNESCO, Education to Prevent AIDS/STD in the Pacific (Paris: WHO/UNESCO, 1991), pp. 16-17.

2

SAMPLE TEACHING LEARNING ACTIVITIES WITH APPROPRIATE EVALUATION

LECTURE-DISCUSSION

I. TOPIC

Nature, Transmission, Manifestations and Prevention of AIDS.

II. OBJECTIVE

1. Identify the causative agent of AIDS
2. Describe the clinical manifestation of AIDS
3. Explain the nature of HIV infection/ AIDS as a sexually transmitted disease
4. Discuss some preventive measures to minimize the spread or incidence of HIV infection/ AIDS

III. MATERIALS

1. Overhead projector/Flip Chart
2. Transparencies or other visuals to present/illustrate: Statistical Data, HIV Modes of Transmission of AIDS, Body illustrating manifestation.

- History
  - *AIDS*
    nature
    mode of transmission
    clinical manifestations
    measures of prevention
- Issues surrounding HIV Infection/AIDS
- Types of usages
- How used

IV. LECTURE PROPER

A. Introduction

Rationale: Magnitude

B. Motivation

- On the chalkboard, print in bold letters the word AIDS.
- Ask students to write on the board what comes to mind and feelings when one talks of AIDS. "Thoughts and Feelings" (Baseline and processing setting exercise)

C. Lecture-Discussion

- Present statistics on overhead.
- Describe Human Immuno-deficiency Virus.
- Discuss AIDS manifestations in man.
- Trace the Mode of Transmission of AIDS.
- Explain preventive measures.
- Encourage questions and clarify issues.
- Synthesize the lecture. s Give a post test of 10 questions.

PANEL DISCUSSION

I. TOPIC

Psycho-socio-moral and cultural implications of HIV Infection/ AIDS to the individual, family and community

II. MAJOR OBJECTIVES

General

Gain a deeper and wider perspective on the implication of HIV Infection/AIDS to the individual, family and community

Specific

1. Interpret the views arsd opinions of experts regarding the topic discussed
2. Share views and opinions on the subject with the panel of experts
3. Acquire skills in the mechanics of preparing and conducting a panel discussion

III. ACTIVITIES

1. Assign students to invite resource persons as panelists composed of:
   a. *Psychologig* to talk on psychological and emotional impact of AIDS on the individual, family and community
   b. *Sociologist* to talk on the socio-cultural impact
   c. *Representative of various religious sectors* to talk on the moral implication
2. Write letters of invitation to be signed by the Dean which should include the time, venue, date and objective of the forum and the expected participants.
3. Prepare budget for the forum which may come from the schools faculty development budget and/or reasonable registration fee to defray expenses for honoraria and snacks for panelists, and handouts and other expenses needed.

IV. MECHANICS

1. Panelists will be given 15 minutes each for the paper presentation.
2. Moderator to be selected by the student body to give the objectives of the forum and briefly introduce each panelist, sum up salient points of the presentation and facilitate the open forum.
3. Open forum may be conducted through direct question from the audience or somebody can distribute paper for any question to be directed to any of the panelists.
4. Secretariat composed of students to collect all paper presentation to be reproduced. If possible papers should be handed in days before the presentation for distribution as handouts to participants. Record all the proceedings to serve as a resource material or ready reference for items needing further clarification.

V. EVALUATION

Sample tools are included for use to evaluate the process and the product.

SAMPLE EVALUATION SHEET (PANEL DISCUSSION)

Criteria	*Very Satisfactory*	*Fairy Satisfactory*	*Satisf-actory*	*Unsatis factory*
A. Process				
I. Venue				
1. Well lighted and ventilated				
2. Acoustics				
3. Physical arrangement				
II. Panelist				
1. Appropriateness of paper presented to the topic				
2. Accuracy of data presented				
3. Clarity of presentation				
4. Authoritative response to queries.				
III. Organizers				
1. Response to the needs of participants				
2. Handouts printing and completeness				
V. Participants				
1. Anendance				
2. Relevance of questions raised				
3. Openness				

EVALUATION ON CONTENT

(For Students - Pre and Post)

Directions: Answer the following questions briefly.

1. Should persons with AIDS be isolated from their families? Why?
2. You come from an affluent family and you have a luxurious lifestyle. Also, you are a civic-spirited citizen and one of your missions is to donate blood once a year. However, when your blood was tested for HIV, it came out to be positive. How will you react to the situation? What will you do?

3. You are an ordinary employee and an HIV positive. Where will you go for treatment, care and support knowing fully well of your limited budget and that your illness has no known cure? What further steps will you undertake?
4. You are an active, intelligent and socio-civic spirited student. And you are aware of the many ills of the country, one of which is the problem on AIDS. How will you channel your energy and intelligence to help fight AIDS?
5. What will you do if you learn that a member of your family has AIDS?

KEY TO CORRECTION

1. No. Persons with AIDS should not be isolated from their family because it can be very distressing and demoralizing. Let us remember that they have feelings and that they should be given the opportunities to express their fears, feelings and anxieties to the members of their families and friends. This is the time that they need moral support from them.
2. Of course, I will be shocked, but being aware of the possible consequences it brings and since there is no one to be blamed except myself, I'll seek professional help from persons/ agencies which are involved in the management, care and support of persons with AIDS. Most of all, I'll prepare myself spiritually so that when death comes, I will be ready to face GOD, my Creator.
3. With my financial limitations, I'll go to agencies, government or non-government, which are involved in the management, care and support of persons with AIDS. I'll involve myself in self-help and income generating projects like handicraft, sewing, etc. These will augment my meager income and at the same time make me busy and self-reliant.
4. I'll get involved in socio-civic activities like organizing groups which will help in the campaign against AIDS and AIDS prevention programs like setting up AIDS information center, encourage friends to discuss AIDS, etc. I'll also help in different religious activities in the church to make me busy and useful.
5. I will be supportive to make him feel loved and cared for, let him live a positive life by keeping him busy and productive.

3

PSYCHOLOGICAL AND CULTURAL IMPLICATIONS PRESENTED BY HIV INFECTION/AIDS ON THE INDIVIDUAL, FAMILY AND COMMUNITY

A. PSYCHOLOGICAL ASPECT

Dealing with the terminally ill, the chronically sick and people with life threatening conditions is difficult, especially when those affected are young. Even those with HIV who are well are often subject to severe anxiety, fear, hopelessness and even loss of self-esteem. Some psychological support for the patient from the family and even the members of the health team and community is essential.

1. Friends, Family and Members of The Health Team

The psychological stress on those close to anyone affected by HIV, particularly if the patient is very ill, can be immense. It is essential that all those involved should have opportunities to express their feelings and fears, whether to each other, to voluntary health workers, or to members of the health team. In many cases, all that is required is a simple explanation of what is going on and straightforward but tactful replies to questions.

Emotional stress should be dealt with as soon as experienced to enable the person to adequately cope with forthcoming difficulties. Advice/counsel should also be sought by members of the farnily.

2. The Patient

It is important for the person with HIV to have every opportunity to express fears and anxieties. The physician counselor should help clarify the patient's sources of fears and anxiety. This may be done by trying to find out how much the person understands his/her condition and by providing appropriate information when necessary. Establishing roots of stress and understanding of his/her condition will help the person and the counsellor identify the purpose for counseling/helping relationship. Persons with HIV/AIDS may require specialized help. There are trained persons available for this.

Many of those with HIV will know a number of others with the virus and may indeed have lost friends, family or lovers. The distress this can cause should never be underestimated. Patients often compare themselves with others who have been in apparently similar situations and, in this case, it is important to stress that everyone is different. Maintenance of a realistic but positive outlook is essential. There are many reasons for someone with HIYto be increasingly optimistic.

An important factor in those who have survived many years with HIV appears to be the degree of understanding and control of their own management demonstrated by the people affected. At all times the physician should explain frankly what is going on, what treatment is being offered and why, so that patients have maximum control of their own management.

Self-help groups and the news letters published by them are a very useful source of information about HIV and AIDS, and provide a point of contact for those affected. Isolation can be very distressing, but some patients require permission to take up the services offered. Every country has groups and organizations providing information and support for people affected by HIV.

B. SOCIO-ECONOMIC ASPECTS

1. Housing

Adequate housing is a necessity for people with HIV as they are at risk of life-threatening infections, diarrhea, breathing difficulties and weakness, and good nutrition is essential. Ideally housing should be self-contained with adequate facilities for storage and preparation of food and with level access from the street.

Social workers can be very useful in pushing for adequate housing and back-up evidence from the attending physician can be very helpful. However, this service has not yet been considered a priority by government. The PW HIV/AIDS own homes have proven to be more cost-effective in so many ways.

2. Employment

The decision to tell an employer that an employee is HIV positive must remain with the individual. It may be totally irrelevant and many employers are still ignorant about the issues around HIV. However, for those who need time off work from time to time for example to attend the clinic, it can be helpful to confide in one colleague provided confidentiality is maintained.

Exceptions are those whose work puts them at risk of infecting others, for example, dentists and surgeons. For these people, there are recommendations from their government/associations or unions which state in essence that it is an individual's responsibility to discuss the matter with an expert whose advice should be taken.

Employment policies should begin to consider the potential loss that result in discriminating policies.

3. Benefits

Government or state benefits should be tailored to individual means and needs. This includes people with HIV infection/AIDS. They should be provided equal benefits as any citizen with any other illness. Benefits apply generally to the individual's specific needs rather than to a specific diagnosis. Someone with AIDS who is apparently well may not be entitled to any state benefits while someone with symptomatic HIV infection may qualify for a number of benefits. Social workers should be asked to help patients claim whatever they are entitled to. In some areas there are social workers who specialize in the needs of people with HIV.

4. Family Solidarity

In families where one or more members are known to be HIV positive, it is useful with the consent of the family to seek the involvement of health workers, psychiatrists, psychologists, counselors and social workers at an early stage. This helps build up trust and confidence which is imporlant as it is likely that the family will need increasing support as time goes on. The principles of care are no different from those for any other family affected by chronic illness and here again the health team is well- equipped to help but the specific issues raised by HIV must be understood by everyone involved.

If problems arise at school, one key worker (e.g. counselor, psychiatrist) well acquainted with the facts about HIFcan be invaluable.

5. Family Expenses/Budget

The basic advice on diet is to encourage a well-balanced healthy diet containing appropriate proportions of protein, carbohydrates and fat and plenty of vitamins. People who have AIDS are usually encouraged to eat when they're hungry not necessarily confining themselves to particular meal time.

For those with chronic diarrhea, ingestion of essential vitamins and minerals is essential and it may be necessary to prescribe these. Specifically food supplement can be a useful adjunct for those with anorexia. Some physicians may prescribe multi- vitamins supplements.

Aside from the diet and dietary supplements, the person with AIDS needs adequate medication. Regular consultation and regular check-up coupled with counselling services are essential. For serious cases, prolonged hospitalization might be needed. All of these needs call for additional financial burden to the family budget.

C. MORAL AND CULTURAL ASPECTS

AIDS prevention education programme must take into account the culture, sexual behaviour and educational norms. It needs to take into account religious and cultural outlook of the community in which the program will be implemented. A basic programme may be designed centrally and altered in each community to make it culturally appropriate. However, any alteration must not lead to the exclusion of essential information and activities.

In the Philippines where there is a variety of cultures or marked differences between urban or rural areas cultural and community concern must be taken into consideration. It is important to create a program that takes into account the customs and culture of the community and to base it on a realistic assessment of risk behaviour (e.g. machismo, feminism) and situations that arise in the community. For example, a community where there is significant amount of sexual activity among unmarried young people, it is unrealistic to promote monogamy and celibacy as the only options for prevention.

Certain cultural practices and norms have pushed men and women to further risk of HIV infection. Thus, it is imperative to examine how best certain traditions can be used to prevent the spread of the disease.

SITUATIONAL STUDIES

Concept: The formation of good habits, correct attitudes, values and behaviour toward sex will prevent HIV Infection/AIDS. These can eventually lead to a more productive and satisfying life.

Instructions: Read and analyze the following situations. Tell if you agree or disagree and why.

Situation 1

Jose, a 2nd year electrical engineering student, is a member of a fraternity in his university. He has been going around with a particular girl known to most of his fraternity brothers. During class breaks, they eat together and engage in conversation on topics of great interest to the group. One day the group talked about their experiences with girls. Almost all of them have girlfriends and had experienced sex except Jose. The group started encouraging Jose to have sex with his girlfriend. They reckon he's not man enough if he won't do what they say. Every time the group see each other during the break periods, the group would be teasing and putting a lot of pressure on Jose to have sex with his girlfriend. However, Jose and his girlfriend have decided not to be sexually involved yet.

Situation 2

Josephine comes from a conservative family where sex is taboo. Her mother and father are too busy with their family business; hence, they have no time to talk to her especially on matters concerning sexual behaviour.

Josephine has a boyfriend and they have been dating almost every weekend. They enjoy going to the movies, discos, and dinner dates. They engage in heavy petting that they become more and more sexually aware of each other. One night, Josephine consented to sleep with her boyfriend.

Situation 3

Antonio belongs to a group of married men who enjoy going to "sex shows" and "beer houses" and pay to have sex with call girls. However, Antonio is well-informed about the seriousness of AIDS. He knows that this disease can be transmitted through sexual contact especially with someone who has multiple sex partners. Such knowledge helped Antonio to say "No" to the group, unmindful of being ostracized.

Note To The Teacher: Similar situations can be created by the students themselves instead of the teacher providing the situations, thus provide relevance and a wide-range of experiences that are realistic.

SAMPLE ATTITUDE SCALE FOR ASSESSiNG BEHAVIOUR

Directions: Below are some statements regarding certain attitudes, values and proper sex behaviour related to AIDS. Check the column which corresponds to your opinion.

SA - Strongly Agree
A- Agree
SD - Strongly Disagree
D - Disagree
U - Uncertain

	SA	A	SD	D	U
1. Having sex experience is a sign of manliness.					
2. HIV/ AIDS cannot be transmitted through only one sexual contact.					
3. It is good and safe to have sex with your boyfriend/girlfriend so long as it is with mutual consent.					
4. It is morally good and safe to indulge in sexual contact provided a condom is used by men.					
5. To be considered "in", one should also indulge in unacceptable sexual behaviour of the "barkada".					
6. One must say "No" to sex even if he will be ostracized by his peer group/ "barkada".					
7. For woman to become popular with men, she should give in to their sexual desires.					
8. If one has problems regarding sexual behaviours, the right person to seek advice from is either one of his parents or counsellor.					
9. It is a wise decision to postpone sexual experience with your fiancee until marriage.					
10. Sexual experiences/contacts outside marriage may lead to unpleasant psychosocial situations as well as the risk of HIV infection/AIDS.					

SOCIO-DRAMA

Title:	Counseling a student detected HIV positive
Objective:	To demonstrate beginning skills in counseling HIV positive individual
Characters:	Teacher and Client
Setting:	Faculty Room Table for faculty and a chair fronting table for client

Dialogue

Teacher:	Good Morning Fe You look heavily burdened. Is anything worrying you? Do you want to talk about it? Sit down.
Fe:	Ma'am (on the verge of tears). My family is intending to migrate to the United States, so we were required to undergo complete physical examination and I was found HIV positive. As I gathered from your lecture last month, it can be possible later on that I can develop AIDS. What will I do?
Teacher:	Have you talked this over with your family?
Fe:	The Doctor talked to us and informed us that this may cause disapproval of our immigration visa. I'm so ashamed and afraid. Not only because I am the cause of my family's change of plans to migrate, but also I do not know what to do now until I develop AIDS.
Teacher:	It's understandable to feel the way you do, but be thankful that you have a family who loves you. I think, Fe, that you should have professional help. Would you like that? The AIDS Unit of the Department of Health helps people with HIV. The Remedios AIDS Foundation is another. They will tell you everything that you need to know about your condition. They can provide you tremendous help which we can't. What is more important, they treat people with HIV with confidentiality. Maybe a relative can take you there. If no one can but you want to consult them, let me know. I will take you there. Talk it over with your parents and tell me what you decide. And, Fe, I'm glad you came to me. This is just between the two of us.
Fe:	Thank you very much Ma'am. I know I can confide in you. Talking to you has made me feel better already.
Teacher:	I'm glad, Fe.

OBSERVATION CHECKLIST FOR SOCIO DRAMA INDICATORS

Indicators	*5*	*4*	*3*	*2*	*1*
1. Greats client with smiles.					
2. Calls client by first name/nickname.					
3. Offers chair to make client feel comfortable.					
4. Shows interest by putting aside work at hand.					
5. Provides privacy by closing door.					
6. Encourages client to talk by listening attentively.					
7. Encourages eye-to-eye contact.					
8. Allows client to talk without unnecessary interruption.					
9. Talks to client in friendly tone and gesture.					
10. Refers to appropriate agency when necessary					

RATING SCALE:

50 - 45	100%	25 - 20	75
45 - 40	95	20 - 15	70
40 - 35	90	15 - 10	65
35 - 30	85	10 - 05	60
30 - 25	80	05 - 0	55

100 % to 75% - passing grade

Note: Teacher can device her own rating scale based on the grading policy of the school.

SURVEY METHOD

Survey is one of the methods of gathering information and data on a particular problem of interest to the researcher. The most common use of a survey is to gather baseline data about your target clientele or population. A very common example is the knowledge, attitude, and practice (KAP) survey. This particular survey gives information/data on the knowledge level, attitudes and practices of your target clientele. Your clientele could be students, teachers, parents, pregnant mothers, etc.

Another example is a community survey wherein information of data may be gathered on a health problem in a particular barangay/

community, misconceptions or superstitious beliefs of mothers on pregnancy and childbirth and related topics or problems.

A sample survey form was devised specifically to find out the available government and non-government organizations or agencies existing in the locality which students can avail of or seek assistance from when necessary. This survey form is a simple exercise or activity for students to experience gathering relevant data on the content of the lesson.

The survey form can be modified depending on the needs of the students as well as the purpose for which this method is to be utilized.

SAMPLE SURVEY FORM

Note To The User:

This survey form is only a sample. The teacher can modify this form based on the needs and situations of the locality.

Name of Community...Date........................

Location/Address...Date........................

A. List down all government and non-governmental agencies available in the community.

NAME OF AGENCY ADDRESS TELEPHONE NUMBER

1. ______________________________

2. ______________________________

3. ______________________________

4. ______________________________

5. ______________________________

B. From each agency listed above, indicate the staff or personnel responsibility/functions .

____

____

____

C. What services and facilities related to AIDS do they offer.

____

____

____

D. How can one avail of their services/facilities?

____

E. What problems have these agencies encountered in relation to their functions/work related to AIDS?

4

STRUCTURED AND SEQUENCED FACTS AND MESSAGES ON HIV/AIDS PREVENTION EDUCATION

MODULE I: CAUSE AND EFFECTS OF HIV/AIDS

Introduction

Acquired Immune Deficiency Syndrome or AIDS is a serious disease which is a global concern. Statistics show increasing incidence of this fatal illness. Table I below shows the global distribution of HIV infection reported by the World Health Organization (WHO).

Table 1. Global Distribution of AIDS Cases
(As of April 1, 1992, WHO Report)

No. of Cases	Continent
Africa	144,863
America	268,445
Asia	1, 442
Europ	65, 875
Oceania	3, 523
Total	484, 148

A more recent Global AIDS/HIV Estimate given by Dr. GEOFF MANTHEY, WHO Technical Officer, AIDS Unit of the Department of Health, is seen in Figures IA and IB.

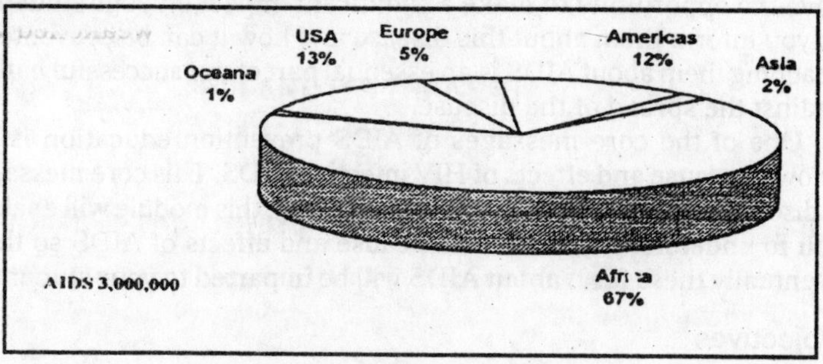

Figure 1A. Global AIDS Estimates

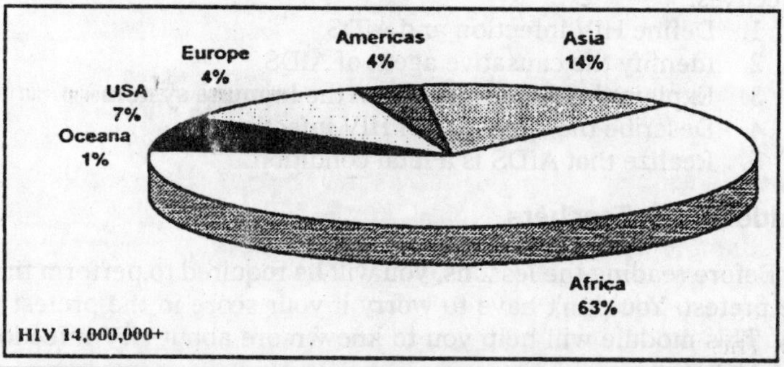

Figure I B. Global HIVEstimates (As of June I, 1994)

In the Philippines, a similar trend is seen in Figure 2. A total of 510 HI V infected and AIDS cases has been reported by the National AIDS Registry as of April 1994. Among these Filipino cases, 367 were asymptomatic while 143 were symptomatic or AIDS cases.

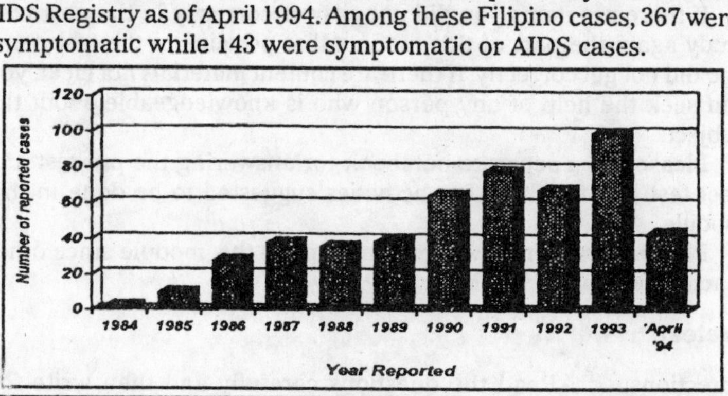

Figure 2. Reported HIV Seropositives by Year of Diagnosis, AIDS Registry, Philippines 1994 - April 1994, N = 510

At present, there is no vaccine and no cure for AIDS and mortality is very high. The only way to reduce the incidence of this disease is to prevent infection from spreading. As teachers and educators, you have the opportunity to make a significant impact on your students as you inform them about this disease and how it can be prevented. Teaching them about AIDS is an essential part of our successful battle against the spread of the disease.

One of the core messages of AIDS prevention education is to know the cause and effects of HIV infection/AIDS. This core message is discussed in this training module. Hopefully, this module will enable you to understand and learn the cause and effects of AIDS so that eventually these facts about AIDS will be imparted to your students.

Objectives

After studying this module, you will be able to attain the following objectives:

1. Define HIV infection and AIDS
2. Identify the causative agent of AIDS
3. Explain the effects of HIV on the immune system
4. Describe the spectrum of HIV infection
5. Realize that AIDS is a fatal condition

Guidelines to Teachers

Before reading the lessons, you will be required to perform first the pretest. You don't have to worry if your score in the pretest is low. This module will help you to know more about HIV infection and AIDS.

After studying this module, answer the post test in the last part of this module. It is advised that you don't refer to the text when answering the post test.

If there are items you did not answer correctly in the post test, study again the part of this module that pertains to the test items you did not get correctly. If there are content materials not clear, you can seek the help of any person who is knowledgeable about the subject.

Please use a separate notebook for answering the pre-test and post test and for the other activities suggested to be done in this module.

Please refrain from writing anything in this module since other teachers will use it for their study.

Pretest

Directions: Read the questions carefully and then write the letter of the best answer to each question.

1. As of April 1994 a total of 510 HIV infected and AIDS cases has been reported in the Philippines. Of these number, 367 were found to be
   a. Asymptomatic
   b. AIDS cases
   c. Africans
   d. Europeans

2. Which of the following organisms causes AIDS?
   a. bacteria
   b. virus
   c. protozoa
   d. fungi
   e. roundworms

3 The acronym for the virus causing AIDS is
   a. CIV
   b. HIV
   c. BAC
   d. ARC
   e. JIV

4. Which of the following diseases results in the weakening of the body's immune system and its natural defenses against diseases and infection?
   a. pneumonia
   b. tuberculosis
   c. HIV infection
   d. gonorrhea
   e. syphilis

5. Which body cells are infected by the retrovirus?
   a. T4 cells
   b. redblood cells
   c. blood plasma
   d. epithelialcells
   e. platelets

6. What do you call the system of cells and organs throughout the body whose primary function is to protect the body from microorganisms?
   a. red cells
   b. lymphocytes
   c. leukocytes
   d. white cells
   e. immune system

7. How would you call those people who have HIV infection but look healthy and well?
   a. HIV symptomatic
   b. HIV asymptomatic
   c. AIDS diagnosis
   d. HIVvictim
   e. HIV convalescent

8. AIDS is a condition of the body which is
   a. acquired
   b. inherited
   c. air-borne
   d. water-borne

9. The time from exposure to development of AIDS is approximately
   a. 1-5 years
   b. 5-10 years
   c. 10-15 years
   d. 15-20 years
   e. 20-25 years

10. How would a person react when he finds out that a member of his family has AIDS?
    a. desperate
    b. apprehensive
    c. angry
    d. calm
    e. sad

LESSON 1
THE CAUSE OF AIDS

(Time: 1 ½ hours or 1 meeting)

MEANING OF AIDS

It is important for you to know more about AIDS because there is probably no other illness of our time that has been dominated by both ignorance and misinformation and because it is a serious public health issue.

You have probably read news items or articles in the newspapers and magazines about AIDS. Are you one of these persons shown in the picture below with questions or doubts on their minds about AIDS?

WHAT IS AIDS?

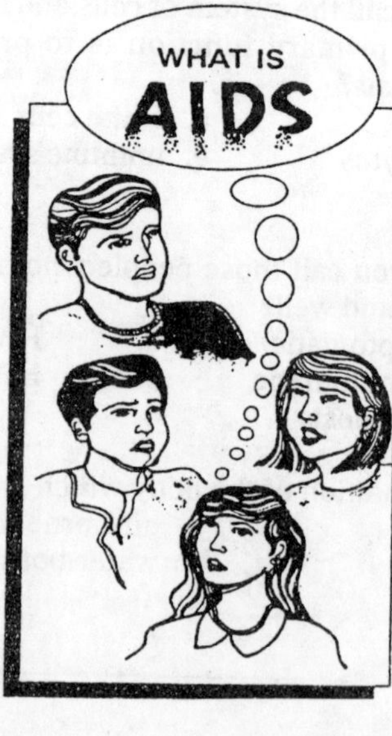

Look at Table 2, Cumulative total of reported HIV/AIDS cases, 1984 - April 1994 derived from the AIDS Registry of the Department of Health. This table shows that more (51%) males than females (48%) are infected with HIV/AIDS. Moreover, majority (68%) of those infected belongs to the 20- 39 years age group. These are the ages of most of our college students like you. It is also very significant to note from this table that majority (75%) of infected individuals got the virus through heterosexual mode of transmission. A few (25%), however, reported mode of transmission is homosexual.

Table 2. Cumulative Total of Reported HIV/AIDS Cases, 1984 - April 1994 (HIVIAIDS Registry, DOH)

* HIV Seropositives	510
** AIDS	143
51% males 48% females	
68% 20—39 years age group 70% reported sex as mode of transmission 75% heterosexual	
27% reported as AIDS Case 58% renorted dead from AIDS	

Legend:

* Includes all HIV seropositives whether asymptomatic, progression to AIDS or as AIDS case; and whether they were dead or living at the timc of roport

** Number of HIV seropositives reported as AIDS case

AIDS is an acronym for ACQUIRED IMMUNE DEFICIENCY SYNDROME. It is a condition of the body wherein its immune system - the natural defense of the body against disease and infection - is seriously weakened. The person becomes vulnerable to diseases, i.e., opportunistic infections which the body would fight off if the immune system were functioning normally.

CAUSE OF AIDS

AIDS is caused by a virus known as HUMAN IMMUNO DEFICIENCY VIRUS (HIV). The illustration below shows a graphic representation of this virus. People infected with HIV may look and feel well for a number of years before any symptoms of AIDS develop. This virus is a retrovirus which infects the white blood cell specifically the T4 helper cell which normally fights off infection of the human body.

Not everyone infected with the virus develops AIDS. AIDS is already the terminal stage of infection where the body is serious]y weakened and can no longer fight the different opportunistic infections such as pneumocystis carinii pneumonia (PCP) and Kaposi's Sarcoma (KS).

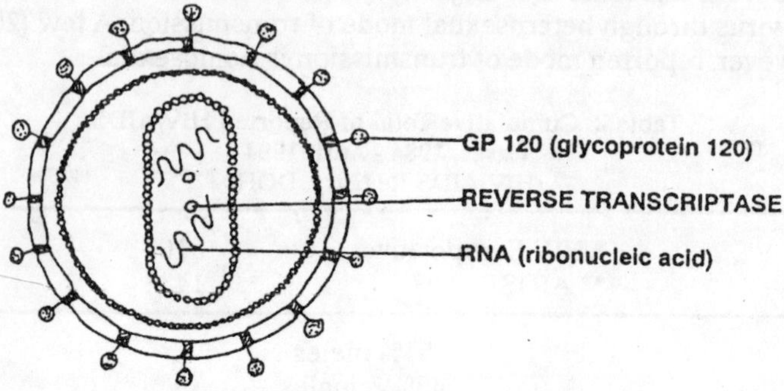

ACTIVITY I. LOOP A WORD

While you were reading about the meaning and cause of AIDS in this module, you came across some important words which are related to AIDS. With the use of the chart below, try to look for these words and write them in your notebook. The words can be found horizontally, downwards, upward and vertically. Try to locate as many words as you can. Check your answers against the Key to Correction in the Appendix.

O	K	D	E	F	E	N	S	E	S
P	S	E	O	T	N	V	M	E	Y
P	Y	F	P	Q	I	R	N	U	S
O	N	I	R	H	N	U	T	W	T
R	D	O	X	Y	M	Z	A	D	E
T	R	I	C	M	D	B	E	N	M
U	O	E	I	O	N	R	S	T	R
N	M	N	D	P	I	T	N	T	C
I	E	C	H	U	U	S	T	P	E
S	V	Y	Q	E	L	A	I	D	S
T	D	C	T	H	C	W	R	I	N
I	A	T	O	V	I	R	U	S	P
C	I	N	K	E	C	T	I	O	N

LESSON 2
THE EFFECTS OF AIDS

(Time: 3 hours or 2 meetings)

EFFECTS OF HIV ON THE IMMUNE SYSTEM

The immune system is a system of cells and organs throughout the body whose primary function is to protect the body from outside attack by foreign organisms such as bacteria, viruses and other microorganisms which may cause diseases if they invade the body.

Human blood contains different groups of white blood cells that play a major role in the defense against disease. One group of these white blood cells is called lymphocytes and it includes B cells and several types of T cells. B cells produce important infection fighting chemical compound called antibodies. Helper "T" cells assist B cells to produce antibodies that fight invading disease causing germs such as viruses. The illustration here shows that first situation (1).

HIV AND THE BODY'S DEFENSE SYSTEM

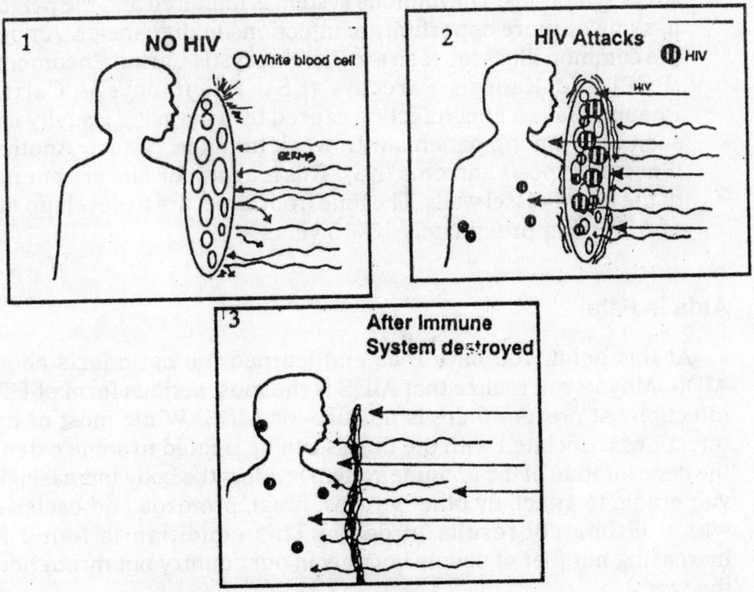

1. White blood cells destroy germs
2. HIV attaches itself to white blood cells,enters, reproduces, and infects other cell
3. White blood cell lose in infection fighting role and poses no threat to germs, leading to infections, AIDS

In Situation B, "Suppressor T " cells stop or suppress the production of B cells antibodies after infection has been repelled. In a healthy person, helper cells outnumber suppressor cells by 2 to 1. Lastly, situation C is what happens in a person with AIDS. The responsible virus infects and kills helper cells, leaving the immune system weak and ineffective in the fight against disease.

Description of The Spectrum of HIV Infection

The spectrum of HIVinfection includes:

- *HIV asvmptomatic.* This appli:-, to those people who show evidence of HIV infection 52SY through laboratory testing, i.e., those people whose blood test "positive" for antibodies of HIFbut look healthy and are well.
- *HIV Symptomatic.* This refers to those people who are HIV antibody positive and who have developed a mild form of the disease with symptoms such as unexplained weight loss, enlarged glands, night sweats which persist for three months or more and neurologic symptoms which are manifested as memory loss and other impairments.
- *AIDS.* This indicates those people suffering from fully developed AIDS symptoms. The immune system is impaired and the person has one or more opportunistic infections/malignancies. Among the common illnesses seen are Pneumocystis Carinii Pneumonia (PCP) and Kaposis Sarcoma (KS). Pneumocystis Carinii Pneumonia is a lung infection caused by a parasite. Usually it is seen only among patients with weak immune system. Another illness is Kaposis Sarcoma (KS). This is a form of cancer or tumor of the blood vessel walls. The time from exposure to development of AIDS is approximately 10- 15 years.

Aids is Fatal

At this point, you have read and learned the basic facts about AIDS. Maybe you realize that AIDS is the most serious form of HIV infection. At present there is no cure for AIDS. While most of the infections associated with the illness can be treated to some extent, the deterioration of the immune system renders the body increasingly vulnerable to attack by other viruses, fungi, protozoa and bacteria, which ultimately results in death. This condition is found in increasing number of people not only in our country but throughout the world.

The following are the reasons why AIDS is considered fatal:

- Once infected one will remain infected for life with the risk of infecting others.

- There is no cure and no cure will be available in the foreseeable future.
- There is no vaccine and no vaccine will be available in the foreseeable future.

The incubation period is very long: 10 years after infection 50% will develop AIDS and only after 20 years 90%.

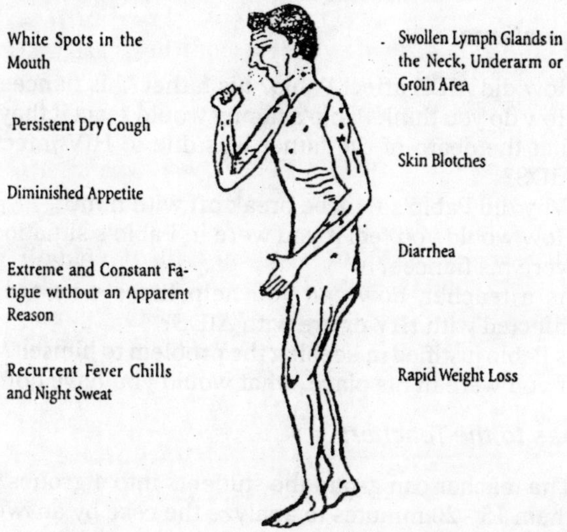

Figure 2. An HIV Infected Symptomatic Person

Study Figure 2. Focus your attention on the symptoms of HIV infection and the various parts of the body that are affected. Describe these symptoms in your own words.

Have you heard of somebody, may be a relative, a friend, a celebrity or popular person who lived with this fatal disease? Here is a case study which describes the effects of AIDS on the lives of people.

ACTIVITY II. CASE STUDY

Directions: Read the case study and analyze it carefully using the guide questions provided. Try to focus and concentrate on the effects of AIDS on the different characters in the case study. You can read the story again if you cannot answer the questions on the first reading.

The Case Study

Pablo visited his father in the hospital. After conferring with the atte nding physician, he found out that his father was positive for HI V. Since he was the first one to be informed, he was frightened to tell the rest of the family. Instead he confided the case to his fiancee who severed her relationship with him. Aware that his mother and his sister cannot understand his predicament, he just kept the problem to himself. So when his father died, they knew that he died of tuberculosis.

Guide Questions:

1. How did AIDS affect Pablo? his father? his fiancee?
2. How do you think Pablo's family would react if they learned that the death of the father was due to HIV infection and AIDS?
3. Why did Pablo's fiancee break off with him?
4. How would you feel if you were in Pablo's situation? If you were his fiancee?
5. As a teacher, how can you help those who are already infected with HIV or are with AIDS?
6. Is Pablo justified in keeping the problem to himself? Explain. If you were in his place, what would you have done?

Guidelines to the Teacher:

1. The teacher can group the students into 4 groups and give them 15 - 20 minutes to analyze the case by answering the guide questions.
2. Each group will share with the class 10 - 15 minutes the highlights of the group's discussion and analysis.
3. The sharing session can be a panel forum with a moderator.
4. The moderator will summarize all the groups' presentations.
5. Conduct an open forum for relevant questions.
6. Conclusion and Recommendation will be drawn by the class and reinforcement or enrichment by the teacher.

POST TEST: MULTIPLE CHOICE

Directions: Read the questions carefully and then write the letter of the best answer to each question.

1. As of April 1994 a total of 510 HIV infected and AIDS cases has been reported in the Philippines. Of these number, 367 were found to be
   a. Asymptomatic c. Africans
   b. AIDS cases d. Europeans

2. Which of the following organisms causes AIDS?
   a. bacteria d. fungi

b. virus
c. protozoa
e. roundworrns

3. The acronym for the virus causing AIDS is

a. CIV
b. HIV
c. BAC
d. ARC
e. JIV

4. Which of the following diseases results in the weakening of the body's immune system and its natural defenses against diseases and infection?

a. pneumonia
b. tuberculosis
c. HIV infection
d. gonorrhea
e. syphilis

5. Which body cells are infected by the retrovirus?

a. T4 cells
b. red blood cells
c. blood plasma
d. epithelial cells
e. platelets

6. What do you call the system of cells and organs throughout the body whose primary function is to protect the body from microorganisms?

a. red cells
b. lymphocytes
c. leukocytes
d. white cells
e. immune system

7. How would you call those people who have HIV infection but look healthy and well?

a. HIVsymptomatic
b. HIV asymptomatic,
c. AIDS diagnosis
d. HIV victim
e. HIV convalescent

8. AIDS is a condition of the body which is
a. acquired
b. inherited
c. air-borne
d. water-borne

9. The time from exposure to development of AIDS is approximately
a. 1-5 years
b. 5-10 years
c. 10-15 years
d. 15-20 years
e. 20-25 years

10. How would a person react when he finds out that a member of his family has AIDS?

    a. desperate
    b. apprehensive
    c. angry
    d. calm
    e. sad

APPENDIX

Key to Correction

Pretest

1. a
2. b
3. b
4. c
5. a
6. e
7. b
8. a
9. d
10. e

ACTIVITY 1 - LOOP A WORD

AIDS
ACQUIRED
IMMUNE
DEFICIENCY
SYNDROME
OPPORTUNISTIC INFECTION
VIRUS
HIV
DEFENSE SYSTEM

Post Test

1. a
2. b
3. b
4. c
5. a
6. e

7. b
8. a
9. d
10. e

MODULE II : MODE OF TRANSMISSION OF HIV

Introduction

In this module, you will learn about the different possible channels by which HIV/AIDS can be transmitted or acquired. Moreover, this will open your eyes to the misconceptions, myths and unfounded fears about contracting HIV, the virus causing AIDS. To make the problem appear real and tangible to you, the status of HIV infections and AIDS cases in the Philippines is presented.

There are exercises for you to perform after you finish studying the various topics. This will help you find out how much you have learned about the topics and the competencies you have gained in the process in order to enable you to advise your students and colleagues who may have fears and doubts about the disease. Use a separate sheet for your answers to the exercises. Check your answers against the Key to Correction found in the Appendix.

Objectives

After going through this module and after completing the tasks required, you should be able to:

1. Identify the modes of HIV/AIDS transmission
2. Distinguish the different myths and fallacies about transmission of AIDS
3. Recognize the magnitude of HIV infection/AIDS in the Philippines
4. Make rational decisions regarding facts and misconceptions about transmission of HIV/AIDS.

Pretest

Directions: Check the blank which indicates whether the statement is a Fact or Myth.

Statement: A person can acquire or transmit HIV/AIDS through:

Fact	Myth	Channels
_______	_______	1. Tears and sweat of an infected person.
_______	_______	2. Kissing an infected person.
_______	_______	3. Holding hands, hugging, touching.
_______	_______	4. Taking care of a person with AIDS.
_______	_______	5. Transfusion of blood products.
_______	_______	6. Donating blood.
_______	_______	7. Sexual contact (vaginal, anal, oral).
_______	_______	8. Mosquito or other insect bites.
_______	_______	9. Sharing food or using dishes or utensils.
_______	_______	10. Sharing personal items like brush, stockings, combs, etc.
_______	_______	11. The mother to infant during pregnancy or at birth.
_______	_______	12. Sneezing, coughing, or spitting.
_______	_______	13. Sharing needles and syringes.
_______	_______	14. Using dirty toilets.
_______	_______	15. Using swimming pools, telephones, showers, etc.
_______	_______	16. Working with someone who is HIV positive.
_______	_______	17. Giving mouth to mouth resuscitation.
_______	_______	18. Blood or semen/vaginal secretions touching the intact skin of another person.

__________ __________ 19. Seating beside a person with HIV.

__________ __________ 20. Talking with a person with AIDS.

LESSON 1
HIV AND ITS TRANSMISSION

(Time: 1 ½ hours or 2 meetings)

MODES OF HIV TRANSMISSION

The virus that causes AIDS, the Human Immuno-deficiency Virus (HIV, may be transmitted or acquired in any of the following ways:

1. Through sexual contact with an infected person
2. Through exposure to infected blood and body fluids
3. Through an infected mother to her unborn or newborn child

Sexual contact with an infected person. By far, sexual contact is the major route of HIV transmission worldwide. About 60-78% of HIV/AIDS cases worldwide were acquired through sexual contact. Genital secretions such as semen and vaginal secretions are body fluids which carry HIV of an infected person. The route of transmission could be through heterosexual (male/female) or homosexual (male/male, female/female) contact. The transmission rate per single contact may range from 1/100 to 1/1000, but the rate of transmission is increased in the presence of co- factors like multiple sex partners, anal contact, STD's (Sexually Transmitted Disease) and other practices that cause trauma to the genilals such as douching, rimming, fisting, etc.

According to experts, transmission of HIV could be due to microscopic lacerations occurring during sex which bring the virus present in the seminal or vaginal secretions into contact with the other partner's bloodstream. The risk of transmission is increased if inflammations, fissures, sores or lesions are present in the mouth, anal and genital areas of sex partners, particularly if any one of them has another sexually transmitted disease such as syphilis or herpes. Since the mucous surface of the rectum is fragile and prone to micro-fissures, anal sex is the most risky.

Exposure to infected blood. Research findings indicate that blood is the most contaminant element of the human body which carries more concentrated HIV than other body fluids; e.g., semen and vaginal secretions. People usually get direct contact with infected blood through blood transfusion and sharing of needles and syringes.

The transmission rate of HIV through a single transfusion of infected blood or blood products is 90% and higher. However, one cannot get HIV infection by giving blood, granting, of course, that the blood-taking instrument is not contaminated. Any used needle not properly sterilized can carry the virus from an infected person to the next user of the needle. The risk is from the contaminated blood that may be left in the needle and syringe. Intravenous drug users are usually infected with HIV through the sharing needles and syringes.

HIV can also be transmitted from one person to another through infected blood left on skin-piercing instruments such as needles, scissors, razors, knives, medical instrument, etc. used in acupuncture, circumcision, tattooing, ear-piercing and others. Likewise, it can also be transmitted during accidents or in the hospitals involving direct contact between the blood of an infected person and a wound or fissure of another person.

Through an infected mother to her unborn or newborn child (Perinatal). Most children who are HIV positive or with AIDS acquired the virus from their infected mothers before birth through the mothers' blood system or during delivery. In rare cases, the babies get the infection during breast-feeding.

During pregnancy, the reported transmission rate of HIV from an infected mother to her fetus is between 40-50%.

MYTHS ABOUT HIV TRANSMISSION

HIVis a weak virus and hard to get. It cannot be transmitted through the air or water outside the human body. A person cannot get the infection from the hugging, coughing and sneezing of an infected person, from insect bites, or from sharing glasses, plates, knives or forks. Neither can it be acquired from public lavatories, showers, swimming pools, toilets, telephones, etc.

Likewise, one cannot contract HIV by being near someone, or touching someone or working with someone who is infected with the virus. The physical presence of an infected person is not enough to pass on the virus.

There is no documented case where the sweat and tears of an infected person transmitted XIV to another person. In the same manner, the usual amount of saliva present in intimate kissing cannot carry enough virus to infect a partner. Lesions or open wounds in the mouth of the recipient should be present before transmission of HIV may take place.

CASES OF HIV INFECTION 1N THE PHILIPPINES

Transmission. Sexual contact is considered the most predominant mode of transmission in the Philippines. About 52.16% of the known HIV/AIDS cases acquired the infection through heterosexual means while 26.23% got infected through homosexual/bisexual contact.

Other vehicles for HIV infection include blood transfusion, perinatal and intravenous drug use (see Figure I).

There are only 368 reported cases of HIV infected/AIDS cases that have been reported to the Department of Health (DOH), National AIDS Registry as of December 1992. However, this does not reflect true incidence due to the silent nature and the speed of spread of the disease, the figure is much more. The above figure shows that HIV infection is hitting the mainstream of the Philippine society. This shatters the stereotyped belief that HIV/AIDS is only for the sexual deviants and drug addicts. The message is clear: anyone, male or female, young or old from all walks of life can acquire HI V/AIDS.

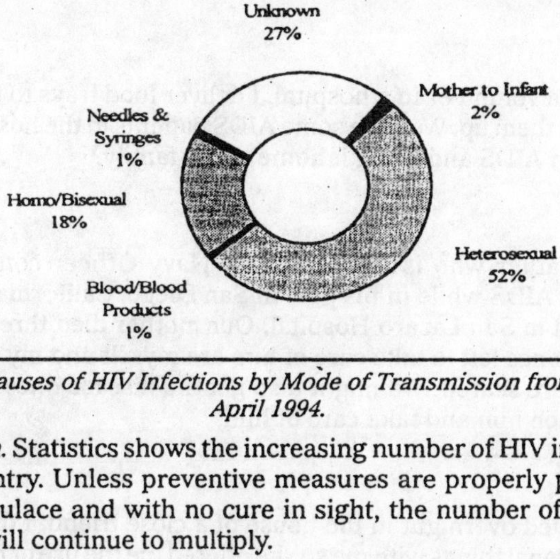

Figure 1. Causes of HIV Infections by Mode of Transmission from 1984 to April 1994.

Growth. Statistics shows the increasing number of HIV infections in the country. Unless preventive measures are properly practiced by the populace and with no cure in sight, the number of infected Filipinos will continue to multiply.

Table 1. Mortality Rate of AIDS Cases from 1984 to December 1992

MODE OF TRANSMISSION	AIDS CASES	DEATH No.	%
Heterosexual	39	28	32.56
Homo/Bisexual	38	26	30.23
IV Drug Use	0	0	0
Blood Transfusion	3	3	3.49
Perinatal	1	0	1. 16
Unknown	2	2	3.49
TOTAL	86	61	70. 93

Mortality rate. AIDS is fatal and it has no known cure at the moment. Sixty-eight percent of the 72 Filipinos who developed AIDS died from its complications. It is expected that the remaining number and those HIV positive who will develop AIDS will also die in a few years time.

EXERCISE 1- Case Study/Decision Making

Here are cases to study. Provide appropriate advice to your students with real or imagined problems about HIV.

Letter 1

I became worried when I found out that my brother is a drug addict, knowing that drug addicts can get HIV infection. My brother lives in my house. Do you think I have AIDS?

Letter 2

I am a volunteer in a hospital. I deliver food trays to the patients and pick them up. We have some AIDS patients in the hospital. Could I develop AIDS and bring it home to my family?

Letter 3

My father who is a retired U.S. Navy Officer contracted the dreaded AIDS while in his post in San Diego, California. He is now confined in San Lazaro Hospital. Our mother died three years ago and the ones left to take care of him are myself and my older sister. But we are scared. We might also get the disease once we go near him, touch him and take care of him.

Letter 4

I stayed overnight in the house of a close friend. I did not bring any personal things with me so she offered me the use of her personal belongings. We ate some fingerfoods from a common tray and later watched x- rated tape. While we were in school, she intimated to me that she is an HIV positive. I hated her for not telling me the truth earlier. Will I get the disease from our casual contacts?

Letter 5

I toured 6 Asian countries as a prize I got from my parents for graduating magna cum laude. I slept with a woman in every country I visited. It was only the other day that I accidentally read an article about AIDS. Now I am very much worried. Do you think I have AIDS?

Letter 6

A reliable source informed me that my classmate in PE whom I share a locker with for about a semester has a positive result in HIV antibody test. Do you think I may carry the virus by now? I am very much worried about this

Letter 7

I had a date with a very good looking giri yesterday. I must tell you that we really had fun hugging, kissing, petting and all those heavy stuffs short of sex. Now, what is nagging me is the question: "What if she is HIV positive?" My friend told me that you cannot tell from one's physical appearance if he/she has HIV.

Letter 8

Last month, I had a blood transfusion in one of the hospitals in Angeles City. I was informed that not all the blood collected for transfusion is properly screened and that some AIDS cases happened in that city. I am deeply worried.

EXERCISE 2 - Essay

Write a short essay on:

1) Who can develop AIDS?
2) Some behaviours/practices that might put the school community at risk of HIV infection.

You are now through studying the module and are ready to answer the post test that follows.

POST-TEST

Directios: Fill in the blank which indicates whether the statement is a Fact or Myth.

Statement: A person can acquire or transmit HIV/AIDS through:

Fact	Myth	Channels
________	________	1. Tears and sweat of an infected person.
________	________	2. Kissing an infected person.
________	________	3. Holding hands, hugging, touching.
________	________	4. Taking care of a person with AIDS.
________	________	5. Transfusion of blood products.
________	________	6. Donating blood.
________	________	7. Sexual contact (vaginal, anal, oral).

__________ __________ 8. Mosquito or other insect bites.

__________ __________ 9. Sharing food or using dishes or utensils.

__________ __________ 10. Sharing personal items like brush, stockings, combs, etc.

__________ __________ 11. The mother to infant during pregnancy or at birth.

__________ __________ 12. Sneezing, coughing, or spitting.

__________ __________ 13. Sharing needles and syringes.

__________ __________ 14. Using dirty toilets.

__________ __________ 15. Using swimming pools, telephones, showers, etc.

__________ __________ 16. Working with someone who is HIV positive.

__________ __________ 17. Giving mouth to mouth resuscitation.

__________ __________ 18. Blood or semen/vaginal secretions touching the intact skin of another person.

__________ __________ 19. Seating beside a person with HIV.

__________ __________ 20. Talking with a person with AIDS.

APPENDIX

Key to Correction

I. Pretest

1. Myth	11. Fact
2. Myth	12. Myth
3. Myth	13. Fact
4. Myth	14. Myth
5. Fact	15. Myth
6. Myth	16. Myth

7. Fact	17. Myth
8. Myth	18. Myth
9. Myth	19. Myth
10. Myth	20. Myth

Ii. EXERCISE I - Case Study/Decision Making

Your advice should approximate the following message:

1. You are not at risk just because your brother is using drugs. The virus is not spread by casual contact. Instead, help your brother get away from the drugs he is addicted to through counseling, therapy, medication, etc. Tell him that his drug use puts him at high risk of acquiring HIV infection/AIDS. Urge your brother to undergo the HIV antibody test so that you are sure about the HIV status of your brother and you will stop being worried and scared.
2. Since the food trays will not be contaminated with the body fluids (semen, blood and vaginal secretions) that transmit the virus from one person to another, you need not be afraid. However, so that you can be really safe, practice the precautionary measures in handling used eating utensils to prevent the spread of many other disease causing germs in the hospital setting.
3. You cannot get HIV infection by casual contacts. It is at this very moment that your brother needs your love, support and care. Give these to him without reservations, precautionary measures should be observed in some cases.
4. There is no need for you to worry. Personal belongings such as towel, comb, soap, etc. and casual contacts cannot spread the virus. However, if you really want to be sure and get away from your fear, go to the Center and get some information about HIV infection and AIDS. There are other centers in the community which can provide additional information or services on the subject.
   What you can do now is to understand and be kind to your friend. I know that you still care for her after all. Advise her to seek counselling.
5. You really have a reason to worry because HIV infection can be acquired through sexual contact. To allay your fear, go to the center and have yourself to be counselled and tested.
6. You have no reason to worry. Sharing a locker will not cause the virus to be transmitted. HIV is spread by the exchange of any of the three body fluids: semen, blood and vaginal secretions. But your fear is very normal.
7. Don't worry. If you are really telling the truth that there was no sexual contact that happened, then you cannot get HIV, even if

she is positive. The virus can only be transmitted by the exchange of body fluids like semen and vaginal secretions during sexual intercourse.

8. You really have good reason to worry. HIV can be transmitted through blood transfusion and through an infected needle. If you really have doubts about your health status, you can go to the Center for counselling and HIV antibody testing. The result of the test is the only thing that can give you peace of mind.

III. EXERCISE 2 - Essay

1. Anybody regardless of sex, age, socio-economic background, religion, sexual preference, etc. (see statistical data) can get AIDS.
2. Some behaviours/practices that might put the school community at risk of HIV infection:
    - Cases of drug addiction in the school
    - Sexual practices among students and school personnel
    - Unsanitary practices in the medical clinic, e.g. unsterilized needles, syringes and other instruments.

IV. POST TEST

1. Myth	6. Myth	11. Fact	16. Myth
2. Myth	7. Fact	12. Myth	17. Myth
3. Myth	8. Myth	13. Fact	18. Myth
4. Myth	9. Myth	14. Myth	19. Myth
5. Fact	10. Myth	15. Myth	20. Myth

MODULE 3: HIV/AIDS AND ITS PREVENTION

Introduction

As of today, there is no known cure for AIDS. Thus, it is very important that you and every member of the society should know the preventive measure to stop HIV from spreading. As teachers, you can inform, guide and encourage your students to practice the suggested measures on HIV/AIDS prevention as discussed in this module.

There are exercises for you to perform after you finish reading the topics. This will help you find out how much you have learned. Should there be difficult items in the test you can always go back to the material. You may also consult medical experts or AIDs educators/ counsellors should you need to enrich your knowldge on the subject.

Please write your answers on a separate sheet of paper. Check your answers against the Key to Correction found in the Appendix.

Objectives

After going through this module and after completing the tasks required, you should be able to:

1. Identify the ways and the means to prevent the transmission of HIV.
2. Discuss what the preventive measures can do and cannot do.

Pretest

Directions: Answer briefly

1. Enumerate three measures to check the spread of HIV/AIDS.
2. HIV can be transmitted through infected blood left on skin-piercing instruments. Name three ways to avoid infection through this manner.

LESSON I
HIV/AIDS AND ITS PREVENTION

(Time: I 1/2 hours or 2 meetings)

As mentioned earlier, at the moment, there is no known cure for AIDS. This being the case, the most that the people can do is to prevent or, at least, check the rapid spread of this dreaded disease.

Basically, the spread of HIV can be prevented or checked through the following measures:

1. Practicing "safer" sex
2. Avoiding direct contact or exposure to infected body fluids, e.g., blood, penile/vaginal discharges or secretions
3. Avoiding pregnancy if HIV positive
4. Maintaining good health and healthy habits

Practicing "safer" sex. Body fluids, including semen and vaginal secretions, of an infected person carry HIV. Precautionary measures should therefore be practiced to prevent HIV infection through sexual contact.

The following are guides to safer sex:

1) Abstain from sex or practice celibacy.
2) Abstain from sexual contact (vaginal, anal, oral) until ready to establish a mutually monogamous relationship within the context of marriage.

3) Prefer exclusive relations with one partner to reduce the risk.
4) Avoid sexual contact with a person who has multiplicity of partners.
5) Avoid sexual contact with anyone who is infected or, better still, avoid sexual contact with a person whose HIV status is not known.
6) Unless one definitely knows that the sex partner is not infected, practice safer sex.
7) REMEMBER that an apparently healthy person can transmit HIV.

Avoiding direct contact or exposure to infected blood and bodyfluids. The three important means to avoid exposure to infected blood and body fluids are: I) screening of blood for transfusion, 2) using clean and safe needles and other skin-piercing instruments, and 3) application of unusual precautionary measures.

A) Screening of Blood For Transfusion

Blood transfusion has a very high transmission rate of HIV (90% and up). As such, one of the most important means to prevent HIV transmission is to ensure that the blood supply is not contaminated.

In the Philippines, the Department of Health (DOH) has been conducting blood screening or HIV antibody testing of blood donors and donated blood since 1987. All blood which tests positive of HIV antibodies is not used for transfusion or for blood products. However, due to high cost of testing, extensiveness of the geographical areas to be covered, inadequate number of personnel involved, and limited laboratory capabilities, blood screening has been confined to few strategic places in some big government and private hospitals. In 1991, about 40% of the blood supply in the country's blood bank has been screened or tested for HIV antibody.

HIV ANTI BODY TEST RESULTS

What is the meaning of HIV antibody test results? Briefly stated, the test indicates the presence or absence of antibodies to HIV. Antibodies are special proteins which the body produces when it comes into contact with a toxin or a foreign substance (antigen). Antibodies are capable of neutralizing, hence creating immunity to specific antigens.

A positive test result indicates that an individual has produced antibodies in response to infection by HIV or a similar virus at some time in the past. However, interpretation of a positive test result is limited. It can mean any of the following:

1. A positive test result means that the person has been exposed to HIV, the virus causing AIDS.
2. A positive test result can not say whether the person with HIV exposure has AIDS or when it will develop into AIDS.
3. A person with a positive test result may never have been exposed to the virus. This is called a false positive and infers that there is always a small possibility of infection with laboratory tests.
4. A positive test result will require further testing for confirmation.

A negative test result indicates that an individual has probably not been infected with HIV or has not yet developed antibodies to the HIV. However, a person tested within six months after exposure to the virus might not yet have developed antibodies; a later test might give a positive result. Also, a few people infected with the virus will have a negative test result. This is called a false negative, and, like the false positive, occurs inequently in laboratory tests. A negative test result is not a guarantee that a person will not become infected with HIV at a later time.

An inconclusive test result, which occurs in a small percentage of all tests, means that the result is neither positive nor negative. Inconclusive test results may be due to a number of medical factors that are not related to the presence of antibodies to HIV. A person with an inconclusive test result may request a repeat test after three months. A retest may yield a positive or negative result, or might again be inconclusive.

HIV antibody test results may help individuals in making life decisions. Individuals may wish to be tested if they have reason to worry or to doubt about their HIV status due to exposure to the virus after a thorough pre-counseling with a trained AIDS counsellor. In this way, they can protect themselves, their family and others from infection.

In the Philippines, an individual wishing to be tested for HIV antibodies may inquire from the Department of Health, National AIDS Prevention and Control Program or call the AIDS hotline - 522-34-31 or 59-74-50. In order to prevent wrongful discrimination, the Department of Health issued a strict policy to ensure the maintenance of confidentiality and anonymity.

B) Using Clean And Safe Skin-piercing Instruments

HIV can be transmitted from one person to another through infected blood left on skin-piercing instruments, particularly syringes and needles. Hence, it is necessary to make sure that the instruments being used are safe, clean and sterilized properly all the time.

Some of the ways to avoid HIV infection are as follows:

a. Use new and disposable needles every time the need arises.
b. Avoid the practice of sharing needles or other injection instruments.
c. Properly sterilize needles, syringes and all other skin-piercing instruments being used.

The most vulnerable groups to this mode of infection are the injecting drug users and the hemophiliacs. There is a tendency for drug addicts to forget the safeness of the needles and syringes being used at the moment they are high on drugs. Also, drugs and even alcohol affect one's decisions to engage in safer practices/behaviour. In some instances, they deliberately share needles and syringes to show their brotherhood and solidarity.

There is a need therefore for the total change of behaviour and attitude of this group. The first step is to stop their dependency on drugs through medication, therapy and counseling among others.

HIV(+) women are encouraged to seek ample counseling before getting pregnant. There is a very high possibility of transmitting HIV to the fetus during pregnancy. The babies with HIV die at an early age.

Due to the risk involved, a woman who has a reason to suspect that she is HIV positive should seek counseling and submit herself for HIV antibody test before deciding to get pregnant. Moreover, during pregnancy, the mother should take steps to avoid HIV infection.

Maintainig good health and healthy habits. Some of the ways to maintain good health are as follows:

1. Treat and cover open cuts and sores, the possible entry points of HIV, with bandages.
2. Avoid drugs, alcohol and other intoxicating substances which affect an individual's desire and decision to adopt precautionary measures/safer behaviours.
3. Remember that fatigue and stress coupled with malnutrition or improper diet lowers a persons body resistance to diseases. Such conditions exacerbates illnesses already present in the body.
4. Perform regular exercise.
5. Maintain cleanliness of the body at home and in the environment.
6. Observe a regular medical checkup which will help an individual know his health status and possible vulnerability to other diseases.

Now, you are through studying the module and are ready to answer the evaluation items that follow:

EVALUATION

A. Essays

1) Identify and explain the measures which may prevent or check the transmission of HIV/AIDS.
2) Is antibody test foolproof or conclusive? Explain.

B. Case Study

Case No. 1

I am a poor orphan living in the house of my rich cousin in Manila. My cousin spends for my studies. In return, I attend to his personal needs and do household chores. He used to work in Uganda as mechanical engineer in a government agency. For about nine months now, he just stays at home usually in bed or in his rocking chair. The other day I had the shock of my life when he told me that he is suffering from AIDS. Now I am in great dilemma. Shall I leave him now when he needs me most after all the favours he has given me? If I stay, how can I protect myself from HIV?

Case No. 2

Before my husband left to work in San Diego, California as a service man I was a month pregnant. Four months later, he was sent home by the US government because he was tested HIV positive. He told me that he got the infection from one of the bar girls there. I am six month pregnant and have a lot to worry about aside from financial matters. How can I protect myself, my baby in my womb and my kids from getting infected?

Case No. 3

I want to get away from drugs, but I know I cannot drop the habit instantly. The most I can do is to phase out the habit gradually by shooting heroin in lesser quantity every time and in longer intervals until everything is over. I know I can do this plan, but I fear that before I am totally free from drug dependency I may have been also infected with HIV. Please tell me what to do.

Case No. 4

I feel lonely here in Saipan. I always long for my wife back home. My co-workers told me that I can go with them anytime I want to cure my loneliness. This means hiring the services of a sex worker in the nearby bar. I know that one day I cannot control myself any longer and will heed the call of the flesh. What shall I do to protect myself from HIV?

Case No 5

I am an embalmer in one of the funeral parlors here in Metro Manila. Every day I embalm about ten dead bodies on the average and have direct contact with human blood in the process. Now that we have HIV infection cases in the Philippines, I fear that one day I might have a client with the infection. How I can protect myself? This is the only job I know which can give me a decent living.

Case No. 6

I am a sex worker. Every night I have about four customers on the average. This is the only way to finance my three sisters in college and provide money for the medication of my father who is gravely ill. I am concerned about my safety, my customers, and my love ones from AIDS. What I shall I do?

POST-TEST

Directions: Answer briefly.

1. Enumerate three measures to check the spread of HIV/AIDS.
2. HIV can be transmitted through infected blood left on skin-piercing instruments. Name three ways to avoid infection through this manner.

APPENDIX

Key to Correction

Pretest

1. Any three of the following:
   a. Practicing safer sex.
   b. Avoiding direct contact or exposure to infected blood.
   c. Avoiding pregnancy if HIV positive.
   d. Maintaining good health and healthy habits.
2. a. Use new and disposable needles each time the need arises.
   b. Avoid the practice of sharing needles or other injection instruments.

c. Properly sterilize needles, syringes and ail other skin-piercing instruments.

Exercise I

1. The following measures may prevent the transmission of HIV/AIDS.
   1.1. Practice "safer" sex.
   1.2. Avoiding direct contact or exposure to infected blood by:
      a. Screening blood for transfusion
      b. Using clean and safe needles, syringes and other skin piercing instruments
   1.3. Avoiding pregnancy if HIVpositive
   1.4. Maintaining good health and healthy habits

NOTE: Refer to the material.

2. Not so. (Cite the limitations and the cases of the false positive case result, the false negative result and the inconclusive result.)

Exercise 2

Advice No. 1

Don't think of leaving him. He needs you now more than ever. You cannot be infected just by caring for him. However, be careful with his blood. Be sure that it will not touch your open wound or sore if there is any. Be sure that the needles and syringe being used by the patient do not prick you. They might be contaminated by HIV, it will infect you. Certain precautionary measures in handling body fluids and waste can be taught to you by health care workers in hospitals or centers caring for persons with HIV/AIDS.

Advice No. 2

There is no danger of getting the infection by being near, touching, holding and kissing an HIV positive person. Try to understand him as much as possible. If you can avoid sexual contact, there are other stimulating methods which can satisfy you both. If sex cannot be avoided, use a condom that does not break, leak or slip off. The condom must be applied properly and use it the whole duration of the sexual act.

There are certain agencies or organizations who can provide you with more information on alternative "safer sex" practices and other care and support techniques for persons with HIV/AIDS.

Advice No. 3

You said you cannot stop right away the habit of injecting yourself with heroin. If this is the case, be sure that the needle you are using is safe and clean or free from contamination. Avoid sharing needles and syringes with your friends, or better still, avoid them totally. Techniques on proper cleaning, storage and disposal of needles and syringes can be taught to you by HIV/AIDS organizations in the country. Seek counseling and advice from doctors and experts. They will help you get away from drugs.

Advice No. 4

As much as possible, avoid sexual contact with a person whose HIV status is not known. Try first some other equally satisfying outlets like touching or kissing. If your urge cannot be controlled and you need a woman come what may, then use a condom that does not break, leak or slip off. A new condom must be applied properly and use from start to finish for every sexual act. Never use a used condom. Take note of the expiration date. There are groups or organizations working on HIV/AIDS that can provide you more details regarding this.

Advice No. 5

Your job exposes you to HIV. It is important that you safeguard yourself to prevent you from getting infected. There are precautionary measures which should be applied such as wearing surgical gown, surgical gloves and mask. These must be worn every time you embalm a body.

Advice No. 6

It would be best for you to be well informed on the various diseases you might possibly acquire because of your job. Apart from this, there are organizations you can go to or services you can avail of in this regard. Through these groups, determine first your risk situation and seek counseling prior to any HIV antibody test. There are still a lot more that you should know and prepare for before any test should be done. Testing does not protect anyone from any disease.

IV. POST TEST

1. Any three of the following:
   a. Practicing safer sex.
   b. Avoiding direct contact or exposure to infected blood.
   c. Avoiding pregnancy if HIV positive.
   d. Maintaining good health and healthy habits.

2. a. Use new and disposable needles each time the need arises.
   b. Avoid the practice of sharing needles or other injection instruments.
   c. Properly sterilize needles, syringes and all other skin-piercing instruments.

BIBLIOGRAPHY

Books:

AIDS Prevention Through Health Promotion: Facing Sensitive Issues. World Health Organization, Geneva, 1991

Education for Prevention of AIDS Population Education, Training Kit for Teacher Education, UNESCO, 1989.

Moss, Adrian. HIV and AIDS Management by the Primary Care Team. Oxford, New York, Tokyo, Oxford University Press, 1992

Prototype Action - Oriented School Health Curriculum Teachers Resource Book Unit 1822

School Health Education to Prevent AIDS and Sexually Transmitted Diseases. World Health Organization, Geneva, 1992

School Education for the Prevention of AIDS. Population Education Program Service, UNESCO 25 Regional Office for Asia and the Pacific, Bangkok, 1990

The Teaching of AIDS Education in Asian Schools. (Status Report from 18 Countries) WHO, UNESCO AIDS Education and Health Promotion materials. Exchange Center for Asia and the PaciElc, UNESCO 25 Regional Office for Asia and the Pacific, Bangkok, 1990

AIDS and the Health Care Worker - A Guide to the Problems and Needs of AIDS Patient

Population Report, AIDS Education: A Beginning Series 1. No. 8, 1989

Publications: (Monographs, Pamphlets, Journals, etc.)

AIDS Prevention Program for Youth. American Red Cross, 1987

AIDS Lifeline - The Best Defense Against AIDS Information.

AIDS Com Aids - Reducing HIV Transmission through Education and Communication

Golescent Education: Sexually Transmitted Disease (Module 4) UNESCO Principal Regional Of fice for Asia and the Pacific, Bangkok, 1991

Nustralian Federation of AIDS Organization Inc. (AFAO) July 1991 No. 12 HIV Briefs

Care of a Person with AIDS at Home - National Advisory Committee on AIDS Canberra 1989

"Counselling Makes A Difference." Population Report, Series 1, Number 35, November 1987. (pp. 1-4)

Education to Prevent AIDS/STD's in the Pacific, WHO and United Nations Educational Scientific and Cultural Organization 1989, Revised 1991.

Foundation fo Health Education and Drug Awareness, Manny P. Mull: .ieda

Manual of Educational Research College of Education, U.P., 1987

Medical Current - A Physician's Digest, September - October 1986 Volume Six, No. 5

The Natural History of Human Lymptropic Virus III Infection

Understanding AIDS - U.S. Government Printing Office, 1988

What Everyone Should Know About AIDS, AIDS Education Program, Handout, County of Los Angeles, California

GLOSSARY

AIDS — An acronym from the abbreviation A.I.D.S. A shortening of the full term - Acquired Immune Deficiency Syndrome. (See Categories). A group of symptoms and signs caused by the Human Immuno deficiency Virus (HIV).

AIDS TEST — There is no test for AIDS. However this is a test for HIV antibody. A laboratory test done on a small sample of a person's blood to detect the presence or absence of HIV antibodies. These antibodies indicate whether an individual has been exposed to the virus.

ANTIBODIES — Substances produced by white blood cells in response to antigens. They fight off bacteria, viruses and other organisms which attack our bodies and cause disease. In the case of HIV, antibodies produced by the body are not effective in neutralizing the virus. These antibodies serve as markers for the presence of, or exposure to HIV.

ANTIBODY — Means a person has been exposed to HIV (see POSITIVE Transmission) and that their immune system has developed antibodies to it. An HIV antibody test will give a positive result for the presence of HIV antibodies. The person may look and feel perfectly well but is potentially infectious and can pass the virus on to others.

ANTIGEN Invading micro-organisms (such as harmful bacteria, fungi, viruses, parasites or other foreign matter) possess specific, unique characteristics which are "recognized" by the immune system as alien substances in the body. This ability to "recognize" substances which are strange to the structure of the body triggers a defensive reaction against the "foreign bodies".

AZT An abbreviation for the drug azidothymidine, more recently called zidovudine.

B-CELL A lymphocyte which matures in the bone marrow, and produces antibodies to pathogens.

BACTERIA Often called germs, these are single-cell organisms, visible only under a microscope. They can usually be treated with antibiotics.

BACTERIA Often called germs, these are single-cell organisms, visible only under a microscope. They can usually be treated with antibiotics.

BISEXUAL People who engage in sexual activities with people of both sexes.

CARRIER A person who appears well but is capable of transmitting an infection to another person. Carriers have no outward signs or symptoms of the virus they are carrying but are infectious.

CLASSIFICATIONS From 1988 there is a new classification system for HIV related illness. Manifestations of HIV infection are classified into 4 mutually exclusive groups.

GROUP I: Acute infection (short-lived flu symptoms soon after contact with the virus) before test results show the person to be antibody positive.

GROUP II: Asymptomatic infection (no symptoms), test results show the person to be antibody positive.

GROUP III: Persistent generalized lymphadenopathy (swollen glands).

GROUP IV: Other diseases, e.g., constitutional and neurological diseases, secondary infections and cancers.

CELIBACY Abstention from sexual activity.

CERVIX The narrow lower section of the uterus, half of which projects into the upper third of the vagina. The cervical canal connects the uterine cavity with the vagina, allowing passage of sperm into the uterus. The opening to the cervical canal is called cervical os.

CHASTITY	Most commonly refers to abstention from sexual activity before marriage. May refer to abstinence from all sexual intercourse (virginity or celibacy)
COITUS	Sexual intercourse, making love, having sex, copulation.
CONDOM	A latex contraceptive shaped like a (Rubber) deflated balloon. It is unrolled onto the erect penis to form a barrier.
CONTACT	A person or animal that has been in an association with an infected person or animal or a contaminated environment which might provide an opportunity to acquire the infective agent.
CONTAGIOUS DISEASE	A disease which is transferred by either direct or indirect contact between infected and non-infected people.
CONTAMINATED	Polluted, made unclear and unfit for use, by the presence of infection or harmful materials
COPULATION	Coitus, sexual intercourse, making love, having sex.
DIAGNOSIS	Identification of a disease from an observation of the characteristics and a knowledge of the patients background and medical history.
DNA	Deoxyribonucleic acid, the nucleoprotein of chromosomes; genetic material.
EJACULATION	The discharge of semen from the penis when the male experiences orgasm or climax resulting from sexual stimulation and excitement.
EPIDEMIOLOGY	The study of how disease is distributed in population groups and of the factors which influence its distribution.
ERECTION	The lengthening and hardening of the penis as a consequence of stimulation and sexual excitement.
FIDELITY	Refers to being faithful to one's chosen or given sexual partner(s) and having sexual intercourse only with that/those partner(s).
HAEMOPHILIA	An inherited condition which mainly affects men. The condition involves a reduced capacity for the blood to clot due to a deficiency of Factor VIII. Consequently an otherwise minor accident can be dangerous because the person continues to bleed. Most bleeding occurs internally.
HEPATITIS	There are several types of hepatitis virus which can cause disease in humans. Infection with any hepatitis virus can result in mild illness that is often undetectable. However,

more severe forms of illness, even death, may result in some cases. Chronic infection with hepatitis B virus also exposes the individual to a higher risk of developing liver cancer.

The three main types of hepatitis virus are transmitted differently:

- Type A through the faecal-oral route.
- Type B through sexual intercourse by the introduction of infected seminal fluids, blood and blood products and sharing of needles and syringes.
- Non A Non B and Type B, through infected blood and blood products.

HERPES — There are two major types of herpes simplex virus (Types I and II) in humans. Some herpes viruses cause cold sores and some cause genital herpes. Genital herpes is a common opportunistic infection in people with AIDS.

HETEROSEXUAL — Persons who are attracted to members of the opposite sex and, if they have sex, do so exclusively with an opposite-sex partner.

HIV — Human Immunodeficiency Virus. The virus which causes AIDS and renders the human immune system deficient and unable to resist opportunistic infections. Sometimes in this manual the words AIDS virus are used to mean HIV. HIV is more scientifically correct.

HOMOSEXUAL — People who are sexually attracted towards members of their own sex and, if they have sex, do so with a partner of the same sex.

HIGH RISK GROUPS — This refers to individuals at greatest risk of developing a particular disease.

IMMUNE — Protected against infection by the presence in the body of antibodies against the organism concerned.

IMMUNE DEFICIENCY — When a person's immune system cannot satisfactorily protect the body, resulting in an increased susceptibility to various infections.

IMMUNE INDIVIDUAL — A person or animal that has specific protective antibodies or cellular immunity as a result of previous infection or immunization, or is so conditioned by such previous specific experience as to respond adequately to prevent infection and/or clinical illness following exposure to a specific infectious agent.

IMMUNE SUPPRESSION — Occurs when the ability of an individual to resist or overcome infection has been severely reduced due to drug treatment, diseases or frequent infections.

IMMUNE SYSTEM	The body's defense system against attack by bacteria, viruses, harmful food substances and some proteins. It consists of cells which, among other things, produce circulating substances called antibodies. Antibodies can recognize materials or agents as foreign and then attempt to neutralize or eliminate them without injury to the host's tissues.
IMMUNITY	The resistance usually associated with the presence of antibodies or cells having a specific action on the microorganism concerned with a particular infectious disease or on its toxin.
INCIDENCE	The number of new cases in a survey population reported over a specified period of time.
INCUBATION PERIOD	The time between infection with a disease-causing organism and the onset of the visible signs and symptoms of the disease.
INFECTED INDIVIDUAL	A person or animal that harbors an infectious agent and who has manifested the disease.
INFECTION	The entry and development or multiplication of an infectious agent in the body of man or animals.
INFECTIOUS	A person is infectious when they have been infected with a pathogen, like HIV, and are capable of transmitting that pathogen to another person. In all categories of HIV infection of a person is considered infectious for life.
INFECTIOUS AGENT	An organism that is capable of producing infection and infectious disease.
IV.NEEDLES	Intravenous needles. Needles used to inject drugs directly into the bloodstream. They are inserted into veins.
KAPOSI'S SARCOMA	A rare cancer — a tumor of the walls of blood vessels. It also affects the lining of intemal organs. It appears as pink to purple painless spots usually on the skin but also on internal organs. It is one of the opportunistic diseases to which people with AIDS are prone.
LYMPH GLANDS	These are small nodes which usually contain large numbers of white blood cells. Agents of infection may be gathered around these areas so they become battle grounds. Infections can therefore cause swelling of these glands.
LYMPHOCYTES	A class of white blood cells responsible for regulation of the immune system. Divided into B-cells (which produce antibodies) and T-cells (which stimulate cells that directly

	fight the invaders and stimulate the B-cells to produce specialized antibodies to join the battle against "foreign bodies".
MONOGAMOUS	Where the two people in that relationship confine their sexual activity to that relationship exclusively.
OPPORTUNISTIC	Organisms which cause infection in individuals with an impaired immune system.
PARASITE	An organism that lives in/on and solely from another. Lice, mites and fungi are all parasites which may live in, on and from humans and in doing so sometimes cause disease.
PATHOGEN	A living micro-organism or virus capable of producing a disease.
PENIS	The male external organ of urination and copulation.
PNEUMOCYSTIS CARINII PNEUMONIA	One of the opportunistic infections seen in immune suppressed people. It is caused by a very common, air bome organism which is (PCP) nommally destroyed by healthy immune systems. It is the most common opportunistic infection seen in people with AIDS in Australia.
PREGNANCY	In relation to AIDS, pregnancy is considered unwise for a woman who is HIV antibody positive. Pregnancy may hasten development of the disease. The baby of a HIV antibody positive mother can be infected with HIV in the wcmb, or during birth.
PREVALENCE	A measure of how common or widespread a disease is in the community or population group.
PREVENTIVE	Measures aimed at stopping the spread of HIV from person to person. As an AIDS vaccine is not yet available the only preventive measure is social/educational action. Such action is aimed both at helping people understand and adopt ways of behaving, which reduce the risk of, or do not allow transmission of, the virus, and at setting up conditions in the community which facilitate the choice of healthier behaviour.
PROMISCUOUS	When referring to sexual behaviour it means that a person does not confine sexual activity exclusively to a relationship with one person. The term usually has negative overtones and is commonly used when making critical moral judgments about other people's sexual behaviour.

RNA	Ribonucleic acid. The genetic code contained in the DNA is transcribed into RNA in order to display the coded functions.
SAFER USE	Those HIV needle/syringe drug administration techniques which reduce the risk of transmitting HIV. Safer use refers to intravenous drug users not sharing needles and syringes or any HIV equipment such as water filters and spoons. If sharing is unavoidable, decontaminating syringes with bleach or alcohol solutions before reusing is recommended.
SEMEN	The cream-colored liquid which is emitted from the penis when a man ejaculates. It is made up of sperm and seminal fluid.
SEROCONVERSION	When an individual who is HIV antibody negative becomes HIV antibody positive after exposure to the virus i.e. blood serum has converted from negative to positive. During this process the person may suffer an acute illness. In the case of H1V infection the symptoms may be those of flu and/or swollen glands. Sometimes no symptoms are experienced.
SEXUAL INTERCOURSE	The physical union associated with sexual stimulation, which usually but not exclusively involves penetration of or by, the sexual organs.
SEXUALITY	The total of an individual's sexual make-up. It includes inherited and acquired factors such as physique, attitudes, values, experiences and preferences. It especially includes the feelings of satisfaction or dissatisfaction which an individual has about being male or female and about his/her personal sexual behaviour and sex life.
STD	An abbreviation of the term Sexually Transmitted Disease. Any disease which may be passed on sexually.
SUSPECT	A person where medical history as symptoms suggest that he/she may have or be developing some communicable disease.
SYNDROME	A set of symptoms and signs resulting from a single cause, or so commonly occurring together that a definite pattern is apparent.
T-HELPER CELLS	Also called T4 cells. These are one type of lymphocyte (a group of white blood cells) that helps in defending against disease by initiating antibody production. In people with AIDS, T-Helper cells are so depleted that the immune system no longer fights off disease and opportunistic infections can occur.

TRANSMISSION	The spread of infectious pathogens from one person to another.
UTERUS	Also called the womb. The uterus is a thick-walled pear shaped hollow muscular organ which lies centrally in the pelvic cavity at the end of the vagina. It nourishes and protects the developing foetus during pregnancy. Menstrual material and blood develop here and, in the absence of a fertilized egg, are usually discharged once a month (menstruation periods).
VACCINE	A substance which contains antigen of an organism. In the vaccinated person, it stimulates active immunity and future protection against infection by that organism.
VAGINA	The closed passage that connects the vulva with the uterus. It is lined with epithelium, lying on connective tissue and a powerful muscle layer which enables the vagina to expand easily during sexual intercourse and childbirth. It is one part of a women's body associated with sexual activity. This is where the penis is usually inserted during sexual intercourse. It thus receives the seminal fluid produced at ejaculation by the man. It has its own "self-cleaning" mechanism, and the acidity of vaginal secretions protects it from infection. Also known as the birth canal because it is the passage through which the baby is pushed during birth.
VD	Abbreviation for Venereal Disease. It means the same as Sexually Transmitted Disease. The latter term is more readily understood and has replaced the term VD.
VIRUS	An extremely small organism visible only through an electron microscope. Viruses cause a wide variety of diseases in humans. They do not respond to treatment with antibiotics.
ULVA	A woman's external sexual organs.
WINDOW PERIOD	The period of time when a person may be infected with HIV, but before antibodies have been formed. This period is usually two to three weeks and is rarely longer than three months. The virus is in the blood and may be detected by an antigen test, but an antibody test will be negative.

•••